TRANSACTIONS

OF THE

AMERICAN PHILOSOPHICAL SOCIETY

HELD AT PHILADELPHIA
FOR PROMOTING USEFUL KNOWLEDGE

NEW SERIES—VOLUME 54, PART 2
1964

ISIDORE OF SEVILLE: THE MEDICAL WRITINGS

AN ENGLISH TRANSLATION
WITH AN INTRODUCTION AND COMMENTARY

WILLIAM D. SHARPE, M.D.

Assistant Professor of Pathology, Seton Hall College of Medicine

THE AMERICAN PHILOSOPHICAL SOCIETY
INDEPENDENCE SQUARE
PHILADELPHIA

APRIL, 1964

MAGISTRORUM DILECTISSIMORUM

EDWARD GROTRIAN SCHAUROTH
1888–1954

MAX LUDWIG WOLFRAM LAISTNER
1890–1959

HOC LIBELLUM SACRUM MEMORIAE

FOREWORD

This monograph is a translation, with an introduction and commentary, of the medical and anatomical portions of the encyclopedic dictionary of Isidore of Seville, the *Etymologiae*. His influence, whether through his own writings or through those of such men as the Venerable Bede, Alcuin, Rhabanus Maurus and Vincent of Beauvais who made use of his works, was very great and those interested in early medieval medical history might find a review of Isidore's information on such matters useful. W. M. Lindsay's 1911 text of the *Etymologiae* is followed except in cases where a variant reading seemed preferable and, in such cases, explanation is provided in the notes. The Latin text may be consulted in Lindsay's edition, or in any one of the many editions of the vulgate text. Latin words more or less confined to medical and scientific writers have, whenever possible, been translated by medical terms, and common words by their modern equivalents as, for example, *disseptum intestinum* (XI. 1. 130) as "diaphragm," but *uterus* as "womb." When uncertain as to the meaning, the translator has kept the Latin word and, in certain cases, the Latin and English words are identical. *Vitreus humor* (XI. 1. 20) is the vitreous humor of the eye, but *elefanticus morbus* (IV. 8. 12) cannot with certainty be identified with any of the various diseases now called elephantiasis. Translation from the Latin has been attempted even when paraphrase would have been more graceful, and the translation follows the Latin text as closely as is consistent with intelligibility.

Words in italics are Isidore's Latin as printed by Lindsay, even when another spelling might seem preferable, and no attempts have been made to reproduce Isidore's sometimes almost punning word derivations or to comment on their accuracy. Square brackets segregate words or phrases either considered spurious by Lindsay or introduced into the translation for greater clarity. Daggers indicate corrupt or unknown forms. Latin quotations in the text are cited as by Lindsay, even when garbled, and italic capitals are used for words which Lindsay prints in Greek characters to distinguish these from Latinized Greek words already on their way to incorporation in the Latin language. Greek and Latin words retained in the translation are reduced to their conventional dictionary forms, except for collective nouns and for a few cases where it seemed clearer to use some other form. Other authors are cited in the notes only to indicate the usage of certain words and concepts in Isidore's time, without thereby inferring any necessary source relationship. The commentary is intended to clarify what the translator took to have been Isidore's meaning, in the hope that his conclusions might interest those for whom the book is intended.

In the footnotes references to Isidore's *Etymologiae* are identified only by book, chapter and section numbers; *PL* and *PG* refer to J. P. Migne's *Patrologia latina* and *Patrologia graeca* respectively; and *CSEL* refers to the Vienna *Corpus scriptorum ecclesiasticorum Latinorum*. Other Latin writers are cited by the editor's surname and the page number of the edition cited in the bibliography.

Like any other work of its kind, this monograph contains faults which *multa dies et multa litura* might clarify, and help has been given the translator by many scholars who have been consulted at various times during this monograph's ten-year gestation. He omits naming them since he must assume responsibility for the conclusions and since not all these kind critics might care to associate themselves with these conclusions.

W. D. S.

Baltimore, April 1954
Jersey City, October 1963

3

ISIDORE OF SEVILLE: THE MEDICAL WRITINGS

An English Translation with an Introduction and Commentary

WILLIAM D. SHARPE, M.D.

CONTENTS

INTRODUCTION

THE DARK AGES

After the collapse of Roman Imperial administration and of much of its dependent culture, early medieval man lived in a land again almost primeval, amid barbarians, disease, starvation, and violence. The fathers of the Western Church insisted first upon the establishment of religion and only then upon the cultivation of letters, but Augustine of Hippo and Benedict of Nursia were neither idle visionaries nor missionary transmitters—they founded an era. Creators are few in any age, but the preservation of man's intellectual capital during those years was the work of many men, not least among whom was Isidore of Seville.

Classical language and literature survived, numerous authors were studied and commented upon, and literate churchmen of the early Middle Ages sometimes wrote better Latin than civil servants of subimperial times. Since each generation views the past in terms of its own needs, in this medieval handing down of ancient learning, pagan works were less likely to survive than Christian; practical men preferred geography, history and encyclopedias to poetry, criticism and drama; and often

writers closer in time survived in greater numbers than those more remote. During the early patristic period, arbitrarily from the subapostolic age until the death of Augustine of Hippo (354–430), Christian thinkers evolved a philosophical theology in response to intellectual pagan criticisms of Christianity and to various heresies within Christianity itself. Augustine is the spokesman of this age, standing as he does at the close of the classical and the beginning of the Christian eras. Later the intellectual climate changed: paganism survived, but it was chiefly from the uninstructed within and barbarians without that the Church's difficulties stemmed. With the collapse of civil society in the West, the Church found itself, willing or not, the accredited representative of Roman civilization: Pope Gregory the Great and the Spanish bishop Isidore represent this period.

During Imperial times, changes had begun in spoken Latin itself. Vowel quantities, an artificial device long ignored in speech, were displaced in writing by meters wherein intensity replaced sharpness of accent, and the ancient metrics were superseded by rhythms based on

5

successions of long and short vowels. Morphology and syntax changed apace, and increasing numbers of new words borrowed from non-Latin residents of the Empire crept into use. The complicated Latin passive verb was often replaced by periphrasis (e.g., *sum amatus* for *amor*), and a disintegration manifest by the third century reached its height in the fifth when secular literature was almost devoid of contact, not only with contemporary thought but with spoken language. Lack of originality is perhaps the most striking feature of late Latin literature, and it is chiefly in religious literature that there are signs of life amid pedantic ashes—Augustine's *Confessions* or the passion hymns of Venantius Fortunatus stem from a flourishing literary tradition, and can still be read with pleasure. When Gregory the Great refused to permit the word of God to be bound by the rules of grammarians, he defended the Christian mind against artificial rhetoric, but the Church's assimilation of classical culture kept Greek and Roman antiquity from following Babylonia and Crete into oblivion. For medieval man, civilization was *Roman* civilization, and even as German tribes invaded frontier towns, they came to respect their venerable Roman culture. Often these barbarians became more Roman than the Romans: names were latinized and before long, socially ambitious families found it sometimes necessary to apologize for non-Latin-speaking grandparents.

Except for Ammianus Marcellinus, no respectable historian wrote in the Latin language between Tacitus and the Venerable Bede: popular historical digests remote from the detailed studies of Tacitus were prepared by Cornelius Nepos, Annaeus Florus, Quintus Curtius, Aurelius Victor, and others. The same process went on in natural science, geography, medicine, and agriculture. Such efforts were brief, practical and inexpensive by comparison with more substantial works, but reflected poor standards of scholarship. The Middle Ages learned of classical antiquity not from original writers, but from fourth- and fifth-century epitomes, from the florilegia, collections of purple passages used in rhetorical schools, and from examples of Latin usage preserved by post-classical grammarians. Much of the scholarship of the first six centuries of the Christian era was philological: Fontaine compares it, with some reason, to drawing a will.[1]

ISIDORE'S LIFE AND CAREER

When Justinian, in 529, closed the philosophical schools in Athens, they had long since passed their days of glory. Classical religious paganism was far from dead—Justinian had been *pontifex maximus* and Augustine found it necessary to fulminate against pagan

deities in his *City of God*—but paganism survived in an increasingly Christian world. About 525 Benedict of Nursia established his monastery at Monte Cassino. Cassiodorus Senator, after years of distinguished service as chancellor to the Ostrogoth King Theodoric, retired to his country estate at Vivarium toward 538 to begin when past sixty the career as an educational reformer for which he is now chiefly remembered. Isidore of Seville was born around 560, and in 563 Columban sailed from Ireland bringing missionaries of that Celtic Christianity which, for a time, threatened Catholicism in the West.

Little is known of Isidore's life. His father, Severianus, seems to have been a person of some importance at Carthagena, where Isidore's elder brother and sister were born, but Isidore's birthplace is not known. His mother's name was Theodora, and both of his parents seem to have been Catholic Hispano-Romans—perhaps "displaced persons"—living in a province ruled by Arian[2] Visigoths. Isidore was the second of three sons: the elder, Leander, became Bishop of Seville, the premier Catholic See in Spain; the only daughter, Florentine, entered a convent; and the younger son, Fulgentius, became Bishop of Astigi. Isidore's parents died while he was a child and his education was left to Leander, who entered both his younger brothers in a monastery school. It is doubtful that Isidore was a monk, although he never married and was always well-disposed toward the monks and their educational efforts. There is abundant golden legend about Isidore, but little of his personality is reflected by his writings. He seems to have had few close friends, but he was widely respected, diligent and hard working, a strict disciplinarian, aloof and reserved.

After Leander's death, Isidore succeeded to the See of Seville on 13 March 599. His long episcopate embraced a time when a mixture of racial and cultural strains were first forming a Hispanic culture: Isidore considered himself a Spaniard, not a Roman provincial. He lacked only a few years of being a contemporary of Mohammed, whose faith almost destroyed the Romano-Visigothic culture to which Isidore contributed so largely, but which added to its own heritage from conquered Christian peoples in Spain no less than in Syria and North Africa.

Reshaping an originally Greco-Hebraic Christianity to the thought patterns of Western man, to be done at all, had to be phrased in Neoplatonic terms, the only philosophical language available and adequate to the task. Early apologists set forth their ideas in a manner intelligible to cultured men of the time: in Alexandria and the cities of the Levant, speculation passed all bounds and eventually became the source of many serious and sometimes socially destructive heresies.

---

[1] Jacques Fontaine, *Isidore de Séville et la culture classique dans l'espagne wisigothique* (Paris, 1959), p. 31: "Éditions révisées, commentaires, manuels de grammaire théorique, glossaires et lexiques, cours complets d'arts libéraux: Rome met en ordre scolaire le patrimoine de sa culture, dans une sorte de testament intellectuel."

[2] Arianism denied the divinity of Christ, considering Him neither connatural, coeternal, nor consubstantial with the Father, and was the religion of many peoples, including the Visigoths, Ostrogoths, Vandals, and Lombards.

Some of the Eastern fathers suspected pagan literature as a cause of this, and in apprehension, some Western fathers for a while banned it altogether. The ban, however, doesn't seem to have been very strictly enforced, and when paganism was less clear and present a danger, restrictions were gradually lifted. Although the later fathers distinguish between the *litteratura* of pagan and the *scriptura* of Christian writers, Isidore followed Augustine's advice that the histories of the pagans do no harm when they speak of what is profitable,[3] and read extensively in pagan and Christian writers. His outlook is narrower rather than broader, but like Jerome and Augustine, he evaluates pagan writers in the light of Christian faith and morals. It is difficult to claim that he hated antique Roman and Greek culture: he simply did not accept its philosophical premises. He was widely and well read, but he was not and did not himself claim to be an original writer, saying of himself, "the reader reads not my work but rereads that of the ancients."[4] A true polymath, his interests were universal: exegesis, theology, canon law, ethics, liturgiology, history, grammar, cosmology, astronomy, physics, and medicine.

Sandys notes, "Though Isidore was himself familiar with many portions of pagan literature, the only authors which he permitted his monks to read were the Grammarians."[5] This seems in fact to have been a counsel to young monks during their formal studies, and not a prohibition of secular reading. Isidore's *Etymologiae* and *De natura rerum* demonstrate diligent, wide, and critical reading no less than genuine interest in scientific learning. In his compilations, Isidore summarizes and combines fragments from both pagan and Christian writers to prepare an encyclopedia useful for a large public and acceptable to Christian faith and morals. Isidore is generally hospitable to pagan writers and is certainly more indulgent than, for example, Gregory the Great, but he is always able to distinguish between theological ideas and practical information.

Although Dampier notes, "It is probable that in Italy some of the secular schools maintained their continuity in the large towns throughout the times of turmoil and confusion,"[6] education and the traditions of scholarship came more and more to be maintained in monasteries or in schools attached to cathedral chapters, themselves often quasi-monastic foundations. Priests were needed for the Church and literate men for government service, so that it is in the cathedral closes and cloisters that the first signs of a new growth of learning are noticed. Isidore's influence, as Primate of Spain, was not limited to his writings since he was a man of considerable authority.

Isidore presided over the second Council of Seville, begun 13 November 619, during the reign of King Sisebut, but it was at the fourth Synodal Council of Toledo, begun 5 December 633 and attended by most of the bishops and abbots of Spain, that he promulgated many of his ideas on education and school reform for the clergy, a group which at that time embraced sometime during the course of their studies almost all literate persons. The bishops of Spain were commanded to establish schools in their see cities along the lines of those already operating at Seville, to organize formal instruction for the clergy and to discontinue the apprenticeship hitherto used for training priests. Students were to live together with an older man of good character to supervise their deportment and instruction.[7] Isidore, like Cassiodorus, considered the liberal arts a preparation for higher studies: bishops interested in training priests would presume that theological studies would follow, although individual students might pursue other courses.

Isidore survived the fourth Council of Toledo by less than three years and, for those days, was then a very old man. He died 4 April 636. Amid the worries of a busy episcopate, he found time for a scholarly productivity impressive in quality no less than quantity, and considering the intellectual conditions of the time, the *Etymologiae* are an impressive achievement. Isidore was not a representative of the classical world and he can hardly be called a medieval man: his outlook is typical of that era which stands between and which is properly termed patristic.

---

[3] I. 43: *Historia gentium non inpediunt legentibus in his quae utilia dixerunt.*

[4] Isidore, *Mysticorum expositiones sacramentorum,* praef. [*PL* 83: 209]: *lector non nostra leget sed veterum releget.*

[5] J. E. Sandys, *A history of classical scholarship,* 3d ed. (Cambridge, 1921) 1: pp. 457–458, quotes from the eighth chapter of Isidore's monastic rule [*PL* 83: 877]: "Gentilium libros vel haereticorum volumina monachus legere caveat; melius est enim eorum perniciosa dogmata ignorare quam per inexperientiam in aliquem laqueum erroris incurrere." In fact, Isidore and most early Churchmen followed Augustine's policy, *De doctrina Christiana* 2. 18. 28 [*PL* 34: 49]: *Quisquis bonus verusque Christianus est, Domini sui esse intelligat, ubicumque invenerit veritatem.*

[6] W. C. Dampier, *A history of science and its relations with philosophy and religion* (3d ed., New York, 1943), p. 75, but note C. H. Lynch, *Saint Braulio, Bishop of Saragossa (631–651): his life and writings* (Washington, 1938), pp. 20–21: "There is no evidence that a monastic school, even that of the monastery of Saints Cosmas and Damian at Agalia near Toledo, was doing aught but training its own oblates in ecclesiastical rudiments including Latin. The schools of seventh-century Spain were strictly personal in their organization; a scholar drew students to him. The cathedral school of the Carolingian type, with its growing impersonal complexion, did not exist. In Spain, in almost every case the scholar was a bishop and the student an applicant for Holy Orders. The register of Spanish scholars of the period confirms this: Leander and Isidore attracted Braulio and Ildefonse to Seville, Braulio attracted Eugene and Tajo to Saragossa, Eugene and Ildefonse attracted Julian to Toledo. This type of school is well-named "episcopal school," "bishop's school," and sometimes "familial school," since the students belonged to the bishop's *familia.*

[7] Ernest Brehaut, *An Encyclopedist of the Dark Ages: Isidore of Seville* (New York, 1912), pp. 84–85.

ISIDORE'S KNOWLEDGE OF GREEK

Augustine, by his own admission, never mastered Greek and, as a boy, detested studying it,[8] and Jerome deferred learning Greek until his scriptural studies took him to Asia Minor and the Holy Land, nor was this unusual among well-educated men of that day. An often quoted rescript of Valens and Valentinian, A.D. 376, appointed a public professor of Greek rhetoric at Trèves with the somber provision, "if any worthy person can be found." [9] Greek was not fostered by the early monasteries in the west, and even the most erudite monks contented themselves with such modest Greek as an occasional Biblical or liturgical phrase required. This is not, however, a knowledge of Greek, and if the not unreasonable touchstone of easy comprehension at sight of Plato and the New Testament be applied, competent Hellenists in the western world were rare. It is important to distinguish between those who know Greek and those who know *a little* Greek. This decline in Greek scholarship antedated the collapse of the western Empire, and by the fifth century was so complete that until the Renaissance of the sixteenth century, a working knowledge of Arabic or Hebrew was probably more common in western Europe.

Many correctly copied Latin manuscripts have survived from the early Middle Ages which contain occasional lines of gibberish, sometimes transliterated into Roman characters but sometimes fairly approximately copied in Greek characters, with marginal notations reflecting some such thing as "it's Greek to me," although before that, Greek majuscules were usually correctly written, if without much understanding of Greek accidence. Gilbert Highet has described this, save that the decline in Greek scholarship antedates the Dark Ages:

In Latin, there is an unbroken line of intellectual succession from ancient Rome to the present day: remote but unbroken. We learn Latin from someone who learnt it from someone . . . whose educational ancestor was a Roman. But the knowledge of Greek in Western Europe died out almost completely in the Dark Ages; the few islands of spoken Greek that remained in the West were outside the main streams of culture. It was almost as hard to get beyond Classical Latin to Classical Greek as it would be for us to reconstruct the language of the Incas.[10]

Isidore was well educated by any standards, but this did not include a knowledge of Greek.[11] It is impossible

to conclude from the *Etymologiae* or from his other writings that Isidore had more than what an intelligent boy might derive from a year of high-school Greek: an impression that the language exists, the ability to copy Greek letters correctly and to puzzle out an occasional word or phrase. It would be incorrect to term this an inconsiderable achievement or Isidore an accomplished Greek scholar: evidence supports neither this nor the claim that he knew Hebrew.[12]

ISIDORE'S USE OF HOLY SCRIPTURE

When patristic exegetes read Scripture, which touched early and medieval thought as deeply as it ever moved any Puritan, they found several superimposed levels of meaning. There was the literal sense, *sensus literalis*, by which what is meant is very plainly stated. Then there is a moral interpretation, the "tropological sense," *sensus moralis sive tropologicus*, by which Scripture teaches men through parables and examples how to live. Beyond this, there is an allegorical or "mystical" sense, *sensus allegoricus sive mysticus*, by which Old Testament books foretell events and teachings in the Gospels and in the life of Christ. Finally, there is a sense unfamiliar to modern men: the "anagogic sense," *sensus anagogicus*, dealing with man's experiences in the life to come. The interpreter of the Old Testament account, for example, of the exodus of the Israelites from Egypt to the promised land might have considered this literally as an account of a definite event in the history of the Jews; morally perhaps, as a symbol of the soul's turning from the bondage of sin to the freedom of grace; allegorically as prefiguring Christ's leading the human race to its salvation; and anagogically as an example of the passage of the devout soul after death from the slavery of corruption to the promised land of eternal life. Individual commentators like Jerome might emphasize history or, like Augustine, ethics, but this exegetical approach persisted all through the Middle Ages to color the interpretation of all literature, profane as well as sacred.

Isidore's thoughtful study of scripture is manifest by direct quotation, but more often through allusions to Biblical events and persons. The Latin texts from

---

[8] On Augustine's knowledge of Greek, see H. I. Marron, *Saint Augustin et la fin de la culture antique* (2nd ed., Paris, 1949), pp. 27–46, 631–637.

[9] P. Krueger and Theodor Mommsen, *Theodosiani libri* (Berlin, 1905), 13. 3. 11.

[10] Gilbert Highet, *The Classical Tradition* (Oxford, 1949), p. 13, omission his.

[11] W. M. Lindsay, "The editing of Isidore, *Etymologiae*," *The Classical Quarterly* 5 (1911) : 42, at p. 44, cites as examples of Isidore's uncertain Greek, confusion between ἠχώ and εἰχών (XVI. 3. 4), and equation of κοτη with *incisio* (? κόπτω: XVI. 26. 5; 3. 6). In general, Greek words in the anatomical

and medical parts of the *Etymologiae* are correctly cited, although often evidently from a glossary, preceded by ἀπὸ τοῦ. Fontaine, *op. cit.*, pp. 849–851, discusses Isidore's attitude toward the Greek language and literature, but it is difficult to subscribe to the thesis that Isidore's relative ignorance of Greek was due to Latin chauvinism or fear of Greek heretical writings, and his reference to Isidore's ignorance of Greek as (p. 852) *choquante* seems ungenerous.

[12] Sister Patrick Jerome Mullins, *The Spiritual Life According to Saint Isidore of Seville* (Washington, 1940) argues for Isidore's proficiency in both Greek and Hebrew, but offers as proof only the observation (p. 11) "the close relation between Spain and the Eastern Empire in this epoch would give a man of his position opportunity and reason for acquiring some knowledge of Greek." Her discussion of Isidore's use of Greek and Hebrew sources (pp. 75–78) is equally generous.

which he quotes do not seem to be those of the Vulgate as it is now received and, save for the Gallacian Psalter, the Vulgate text was only beginning to enjoy wide usage during the seventh century, although final decision in this matter must await a critical text of Jerome's translation. It is likely that, like Gregory of Tours and the Venerable Bede, Isidore used both the Vulgate and several versions of the *Vetus latina* and *Itala* translations antedating the Vulgate.[13] Possibly some of Isidore's textual vagaries result from citation of scripture from memory, or from the use of inaccurate texts. Isidore knew of Jerome's studies in the East,[14] but his chief Biblical texts were probably not those of the Vulgate.

NATURAL SCIENCE AND THE LIBERAL ARTS

It is an oversimplification to state that for the Middle Ages, natural science only explains the first chapter of Genesis, but it is an oversimplification which contains a grain of truth. The scientific culture of the early medieval schools was a book science, little concerned with technology. Since directly subject to Latin culture, western Europe had only indirect contact with Greek scientific traditions and, for the most part, little contact with pre-Byzantine Greek thought until the fourteenth century. The Arabs knew some of the Greek scientific literature—Galen, Aristotle, probably Ptolemy, a few of the early medical writers, astronomers, and mathematicians—through translations made by their conquered Eastern Christian and Jewish subjects. The Latin West, during the early Middle Ages, depended upon such scientific amateurs as Pliny, and upon Greek philosophical notions handed down, for example, by Cicero and Boethius. The Roman secular mentality neither assimilated Greek scientific culture nor made much sustained effort to transmit it to the Latin world: the Roman was typically content to take over the findings of Greek mathematics as applied, for example, to bridge building but was unconcerned with their theoretical verifications or bases. Brehaut misses the point when he states that "Roman science was wholly a science of authority, and the greatest scientist was the greatest accumulator of previous authorities,"[15] since Roman and medieval science is always organized knowledge, whether resting on accumulated data or long authority.

What Augustine denounces as science is often astrology, then almost inextricably intermixed with astronomy,[16] and general scientific studies had shared in a widespread decline of intellectual culture. Medieval man tried to explain a universe created by a superior, powerful, and intensely personal Being Who manifested Himself in diverse ways, including the works of nature. Allegory, which Lear calls "as fundamental as the acceptance of the objective existence of ideas, universals, and their appropriate discarnate spirits or intelligences,"[17] led to explanations of physical and psychological phenomena through superficial and sometimes mechanical correlations rather than logical analysis and careful experimental verification. Rudolf Allers has summed up this role of analogy:

Analogy is a principle of the whole realm of being. But no thing loses, by virtue of any analogy, its proper nature. This is true of concrete things and of universals, of existing things and of *entia rationis*. Numbers may have all kinds of symbolic signification, and their relations may reveal others of a much loftier dignity: but numbers remain, nonetheless, modes by which to express adequately the quantitative aspect of reality. The laws of mathematics are as such in no way laws of suprasensory reality; as such, they are just true propositions on the "behavior" of numbers; but they "express" also truths concerning a realm of a very different nature.[18]

Although much early medieval scientific thinking is based on analogies which strike the modern reader as absurd, Isidore and the educational program outlined in his *Etymologiae* share genuine interest in natural science as knowledge in its own right. Dissatisfied with the theologically rethought syntheses of Tertullian and Lactantius, Isidore turned to the best sources available to him whatever their shortcomings, the encyclopedias and epitomes of diligent but uncritical Roman amateurs.

THE ROMAN ENCYCLOPEDIC TRADITION

The Latin literature studied in schools centers on the literary masterpieces of the Republican and Augustan ages, but in science, scholarship and philosophy, law, applied science, and technology, Roman writers largely concerned themselves with practical works of instruction or reference, and it is sometimes unappreciated just how large a bulk of the Greek and Latin writings which have survived consists of quite prosaic material. Much of this ancient philology, literary criticism, lexicography, history, science and law awaits critical editing, is difficult to obtain and has yet to be translated into modern languages. Nevertheless, such material is the beginning of medieval and modern scholarship, it was often the basis upon which the Renaissance built, and some understanding of it is essential for any adequate appreciation of western scientific and intellectual development.[19]

[13] Lynch, *op. cit.,* p. 121, suggests that Isidore and Braulio, like Gregory of Tours and Bede, used both the older *Itala* and the Vulgate texts.

[14] See V. 39. 37.

[15] Brehaut, *op. cit.,* p. 76.

[16] For Augustine's condemnation of astrology, see, e.g., *Confessions* 7. 6. 8–10. Isidore distinguishes between the legitimate study of the heavenly bodies and their motions, and the superstitious casting of horoscopes at III. 27. 1–2.

[17] F. S. Lear, "St. Isidore and medieval science," *The Rice Institute Pamphlet* 23 (1936): 95.

[18] Rudolf Allers, "Microcosmus," *Traditio* 2: 371, 1944.

[19] W. H. Stahl, *Roman Science* (Madison, Wisconsin, 1962) reviews the Roman scientific and encyclopedic tradition and its influence in the early Middle Ages.

The Roman encyclopedic tradition begins with Latin literature itself. Marcus Porcius Cato, "The Censor" (234–149 B.C.), wrote, toward 180 B.C., an outline of agriculture, rhetoric, and medicine for his son: this touched upon military science and jurisprudence to round out what he considered an adequate general education. Pliny preserves Cato's advice to beware Greek physicians,[20] concluding with the famous *interdixi tibi de medicis,* and although Pliny may have known Cato's work on medicine, he does not cite his name as a medical authority.

Marcus Terentius Varro (116–27 B.C.) was the first systematic Latin philologist and antiquarian, and his encyclopedia, the *Disciplina,* was a prototype for many later efforts. Varro depended heavily on earlier Greek writers,[21] and, although he draws upon his own experience and observation, his work is largely derivative. He follows the Alexandrian tradition of literary criticism, obvious in Isidore's *Etymologiae,* and divides his analyses into reading, *lectio;* interpretation, *enarratio;* the correction of confused or corrupt passages, *emendatio;* and formal qualitative evaluation, *judicium.* Language itself, *lingua,* and usage, *sermo,* also came under scrutiny: all these branches of study were included in what the early Middle Ages would call grammar,[22] and all these branches are reflected in Isidore's definitions and derivations of words. Isidore frequently cites Varro by name as an authority.

Titus Lucretius Carus (*ca.* 95–55 B.C.) is no encyclopedist but is the only surviving Roman writer who presents a unified interpretation of the physical universe, although his epic remains poetry far removed from observation or experiment. Whatever his literary greatness, his science is feeble when compared with his Greek sources and is, as science, much overrated—the scientific tradition of Latin literature is more typically represented by the encyclopedias and specialized manuals produced in such great numbers. Commonly thought to have been lost all through the Middle Ages until rediscovered by Poggio in 1418, Isidore read Lucretius as a scientific authority, and occasionally seems to preempt his words almost unchanged.[23]

C. Plinius Secundus (A.D. 23–79), widely traveled and immensely if unsystematically erudite, completed his *Historia naturalis* while at Rome and died at Vesuvius while trying to observe its lava flow. Pliny typifies the education, tastes, and temperament of the well-educated Roman of his day: diligent and curious, he lacked only critical standards. His writings suited medieval tastes and were widely read. Isidore knew Pliny well, whether at first hand or from Solinus' epitime, the *Polyhistor,* itself a very popular work.

Lucius Annaeus Seneca's (3 B.C.–A.D. 65) *Quaestiones naturales* are even more completely borrowed material than Pliny's, but he is more critical. His work serves chiefly to illustrate how rhetorical an approach to natural science can be. Pliny and Seneca were never lost through the Middle Ages: widely and constantly read, at first or second hand, they formed one of the chief means by which ancient scientific knowledge was transmitted. Few medieval men had the library resources or linguistic skill to go beyond their statements, and acquaintance with Pliny and Seneca is necessary for any insight into the development of the medieval scientific tradition.

C. Suetonius Tranquillus' (*ca.* A.D. 69–140) lost *Prata* [24] seem to have been, like Aulus Gellius' (*ca.* A.D. 123–165) *Noctes atticae,* entertaining and sometimes informative miscellanies, but hardly organized encyclopedias.[25] Aulus Gellius deals with philosophy, lexicography, and history, especially with the literature of the Augustan age and earlier. Although his scientific authorities seem to have been the same as those used by Pliny, the two writers are probably independent. Suetonius' *Prata* are lost, and fragments do not permit more than conjecture as to their contents.

The *Satyricon* of Martianus Mineus Felix Capella, written at Carthage early in the fifth century A.D., is a fascinating production. Books I–III are an elaborate allegory, the *Nuptiae Philologiae et Mercurii,* "The marriage of literature and Mercury," in which the seven liberal arts are presented as bridesmaids to literature on the occasion of her marriage, and in the seven books which follow, each presents a résumé in verse of her teachings. The work was popular and, despite changed literary tastes, contains some valuable material. Anicius Manlius Severinus Boethius (*ca.* 480–524) wrote on music, arithmetic, and geometry, as well as other minor topics. He translated into Latin and commented upon the *Categories* and *De interpretatione* of Aristotle, the *Isagoge* of Porphyry and wrote on Cicero's *Topica.* Although now best known for his *Consolatio philosophiae,* his medieval influence was based on his scientific and philosophical commentaries.

Flavius Magnus Aurelius Cassiodorus Senator was born about 490 at Scyllacium, was Consul in 514, Master of Offices before 526 and a Praetorian Prefect in 533. His plans for a Christian university at Rome patterned after the pagan schools at Athens and Alex-

---

[20] Pliny, *Historia naturalis* 29. 1. 7–8.

[21] Varro refers to gloss collections at *De lingua latina* 7. 10 and 7. 107.

[22] Isidore defines grammar simply (I. 5. 1) as the science of correct speech, both the origin and the foundation of the liberal arts.

[23] Three verses of Lucretius (*De rerum natura* 5. 1275–1277) are quoted at XVI. 20, 1, and see below, note on IV. 6. 18. Lucretius is cited, although not by name, as a scientific authority in Isidore's *De natura rerum* 39, where he paraphrases Lucretius' account of the influence of climate in plague epidemics, retaining the use of *locus* for "pore."

[24] There are a number of etymologies among the fragmentary works in C. L. Roth, *C. Suetoni Tranquilli quae supersunt omnia* (Leipzig, 1902), pp. 276–320.

[25] Aulus Gellius, *Noctes Atticae* 3. 16; 4. 19; 17. 11 and 18. 10 are of medical interest, and he comments on the history of the Roman epitomes in his preface.

andria were shattered by the death of Pope Agapetus in 536, but his interest in education continued, and he urged monks and students in church schools to study the standard classical writers, to diligent historical and literary research and, above all, to careful work in the scriptorium. He established orthographic rules for copying manuscripts, but unfortunately for later palaeographers, suggested that emendations be written in the same hand as the text when recopied. A man of wide learning, considerable wealth and unsurpassed genius for organization, he spared no pains to assemble a library. His *Institutes* amount to an introduction to the humanities and divinity studies with suggestions for more extensive reading. Laistner outlines Cassiodorus' library, a monastic library of the best type at the dawn of the Middle Ages:

The result was impressive and, in spite of gaps, a very representative collection. Besides most of Ambrose, Augustine, and Jerome, and the chief works of Hilary and John Cassian, there were many less known treatises and commentaries, such as Primasius on the Apocalypse, Pelagius' Exposition of the Pauline Epistles, or the works of Tyconius. Greek theology was represented by homilies or commentaries of Origen, and small portions of the writings of Athanasius, Clement and Cyril of Alexandria, and John Chrysostom, and by Latin translations of some Greek works made before Cassiodorus' time. There was a good selection of historical works, both pagan and Christian. Philosophy was chiefly represented by the translations and commentaries of Boethius A large collection of grammatical works, but few rhetorical treatises—though Quintilian was among them—some Ciceronian speeches, Virgil, Horace, Lucan, and, finally, some medical and agricultural handbooks made up a library of remarkable richness in that age, as well as one admirably adapted to those purposes which Cassiodorus had in view.[26]

It is impossible to say to what extent Isidore's library resources compared with Cassiodorus', but libraries did exist in sixth-century Europe, and there was effort directed at the preservation of works of scholarly interest in a variety of fields.

LATE LATIN MEDICAL LITERATURE

During Roman times and until early in the nineteenth century, lack of formally defined requirements for admission to medical practice made the limits of medical education much broader than now the case, and obscured the presently clear delineation between physician and layman.[27] Both in ancient Rome and in the west during the early Middle Ages, *bona fide* medical training extended to three fairly distinct groups: medical craftsmen who learned their profession by a practical apprenticeship, and who provided most general medical care; a small but extremely influential group of master physicians who learned their profession through formal study of classical Greco-Roman medical texts with another physician; and, finally, a group of well educated laymen and clerics who did not formally practice medicine, as physicians, but for whom the study of medical literature was part of a general education.[28] It is apparently for this group, and not for physicians as such, that Isidore intended the medical and anatomical portions of his *Etymologiae*.

From the second or third century after Christ, there developed a Latin medical literature accompanying the rise of Latin as a world language and steady decline in Greek scholarship. Latin was the common spoken language in Italy, France, and Spain, and a very widely acquired second language in North Africa, Germany, and the British Isles. This movement was centered not in Rome but in the provinces, and especially in North Africa, where flourished during the fourth and fifth centuries, Vindicianus, friend of Augustine of Hippo and private physician to the Emperor Valentinian; his famous pupil, Theodore Priscian; and Cassius Felix, the last of the classical medical compilers. There were smaller centers in Gaul, at Bordeaux, and Ravenna, where Galen and Oribasius were studied and commented upon much as they had been centuries earlier in the schools of Alexandria. Many of these Latin compilations and translations were done carelessly to begin with, and some have survived in forms so garbled as to be unintelligible, but despite obscurities these works are our chief sources of information not only for the medical practice of the early Middle Ages, but of post-classical Greece and Rome.

Works thus translated, compiled, and disseminated were selected for their immediate usefulness and, when digests were prepared from longer works, theoretical discussion was eliminated in favor of portions of more practical applicability. A new medical literature emerged which consisted of catechisms, letters, and brief outlines on topics of medical interest. These compilations were, for the most part, anonymous, but some were ascribed to the great—medical and otherwise—to lend them greater authority. Medical manuscripts surviving from Carolingian times are chiefly of this genre and, although many were copied in

---

[26] M. L. W. Laistner, *Thought and Letters in Western Europe, A.D. 500–900* (2nd ed., London, 1957), pp. 102–103.

[27] F. H. Garrison, *An introduction to the history of medicine* (3rd ed., Philadelphia, 1922), p. 103: "Besides the 'medici' proper, there were the herb gatherers (*rhizotomi*), the drug-peddlers (*pharmacopolae*), the salve-dealers (*unguentarii*), the army surgeons (*medici cohortis, medici legionis*), and the *archiatri*, or body physicians to the emperors, some of whom were also public or communal (*archiatri populares*). There were also the less reputable *iatroliptae*, or bath attendants, *medicae* or female healers, *sagae* or wise-women, *obstetricae*, or midwives, the professional poisoners (*pharmacopoei*), and

the depraved characters who sold philters and abortifacients. A very dubious and much satirized class were the eye specialists or oculists (*medici ocularii*) who, each of them, sold a special eye salve stamped with his own private seal."

[28] See I. E. Drabkin, "On Medical Education in Greece and Rome," *Bulletin of the History of Medicine* 15 (1944): 333, and L. C. MacKinney, "Medical Education in the Middle Ages," *Journal of World History* 2 (1955): 835.

monasteries, J. J. Walsh's claim that from earliest medieval times these monasteries were in touch with Byzantine medical writers—Aëtius of Amidia, Alexander of Tralles, and Paulus Aegineta included [29]—is unfounded. Written medical tradition in the early Middle Ages, inside or outside monasteries, was as the Romans had left it, in abstract, epitome, and digest of earlier and largely Greek authorities.

Certain works of the Hippocratic collection were early translated into Latin, and enjoyed wide circulation: most popular were the *Aphorisms* and *Prognostics,* to which Isidore refers,[30] but there were early versions in Latin at least of the *De aëre, aquis et locis,* a Christianized form of the *Oath,* the *De septimanis,* and parts of the *De natura hominis.*[31] Although few early Latin versions of the works of Galen (A.D. 131–201) have survived, his writings were a quarry from which a very large number of short Latin treatises were mined, and a Latin manuscript of the ninth or tenth century at Milan preserves some glosses on the *De sectis,* the *Ars medica,* the *De pulsibus,* and the *Therapeia ad Glauconem de medendi methodo,* suggesting that these works were known and studied.[32]

Cornelius Celsus (*fl. ca.* A.D. 14–37) wrote a complete Latin textbook of medicine which constitutes the oldest surviving post-Hippocratic medical text, and which is the principal source for the study of Hellenistic surgical practice. His *De re medica* or *De medicina* was part of a larger encyclopedia, and its elegant latinity was a model for clear medical exposition for centuries. Pliny compliments Celsus by calling him *auctor* rather than *medicus:* Celsus' medicine is of high ethical calibre, sensible and humane. After a short historical introduction, the earliest discussion of medical history in Latin, Books I–IV consider diseases best managed by diet and regimen, and Books V–VIII discuss those best treated by drugs or surgery. Evidence suggests that this book is a compilation from various Greek sources: Celsus was not unknown to the Middle Ages, but Isidore mentions him by name only as a writer on agriculture, much like Columella.[33]

There are references in Pliny to a lost herbal written in Greek during Republican times by Sextius Niger: only fragments survive, and its direct medieval influence must have been slight.[34] Pedanius Dioscorides, born in the Greek town of Anazarba, served in Nero's army, A.D. 54 to 68, and studied materia medica in much the same manner as Theophrastus had approached botany. His *Materia medica (Peri hylês iatrikês)* does not seem, at first, to have been illustrated, but to have been a practical guide to medicinal herbs. Soon translated into Latin, fragments of these early translations may survive as interpolations in the *Herbarius* of "Pseudo-Apuleius" and in the *Etymologiae.*[35] Dioscorides provides practical descriptions of the herbs which usually include the plant's characteristics, habitat and pharmaceutical preparation: some of the drugs mentioned are still in use, among them belladonna, colchicum, hyoscyamus and opium. The "Pseudo-Apuleius" herbal evolved by the fifth or sixth century, and is antedated by a fourth century, or earlier, Latin version of Dioscorides to which is often attached a treatise on the herb betony, *De herba vettonica,* attributed to Antonius Musa, physician to Augustus Caesar and dead several centuries before it appeared. A shorter compilation, the *Liber Dioscoridis de herbis femininis,* probably represents a differing line of textual descent from Dioscorides, and describes some medicinal herbs, omitting animal and mineral drugs, together with notations of their clinical use.[36] These herbals were intended as practical manuals for practicing physicians, and contained little magical material.

Although the art of drawing from nature seems to have declined very early in the Middle Ages, the illustrations of plants complete with leaves, flowers, and roots incorporated in these herbals were important aids to identification of free growing species, a problem complicated by lack of a systematic scientific nomenclature. The quality of these illustrations gradually deteriorated with repeated copying, but were nevertheless reproduced as woodcuts with the first printed herbals. Later in the Middle Ages, by the tenth or eleventh century, an alphabetical version of this herbal became popular and, with the adscription of still more parts and descriptions, a widely used, illustrated manual of materia medica evolved.[37]

Scribonius Largus, about A.D. 47, wrote *On the composition of drugs (Compositiones = "prescriptions")* outlining not only his own pharmacological views but many of those of his predecessors, arranged by the symptoms or diseases for which they were recommended. The book was intended for laymen as well as physicians, and although it includes most of the score or so of ancient drugs with predictable pharmacologic effect, it embraces many of the wonderful remedies such as hyena bile and desiccated crocodile

---

[29] J. J. Walsh, *Medieval Medicine* (London, 1920), pp. 26–27.

[30] IV. 10. 1–2.

[31] On Latin translations of Hippocrates, see H. E. Sigerist, "The Latin Medical Literature of the Early Middle Ages," *Journal of the History of Medicine* 13 (1958) : 133, and Pearl Kibre, "Hippocratic Writings in the Middle Ages," *Bulletin of the History of Medicine* 18 (1945) : 371.

[32] Codex Ambrosianus G108.

[33] XVII. 1. 1.

[34] Pliny, *Historia naturalis* I. 12. 33–34; fragments in Max Wellman, *Dioskurides* (Berlin, 1914) 3: pp. 146–148.

[35] Sigerist, *op. cit.,* p. 132.

[36] Codex Harleianus 4986 (f. 44R) describes the work: *libellum botanicum ex dioscoridis libris in latinum sermonem conversum in quo depicte sunt herbarum figure,* published by H. F. Kästner, "Pseudo-Dioscorides de herbis femininis," *Hermes* 31 (1896) : 578–636.

[37] The question is thoroughly reviewed by Charles Singer, "The Herbal in Antiquity," *Journal of Hellenic Studies* 47 (1927) : 1.

testes which glutted pharmacopeias until the nineteenth century. Though Scribonius wrote at a time not far removed from silver latinity, his style is crude and since his approach to medicine is that of a cookbook, his contribution to our understanding of ancient medicine is meager.

"Quintus Serenus Sammonicus" seems to have been a third-century father and son contemporaneous with the Severines who wrote a *Liber medicinalis* in hexameter, based on Pliny and other literary sources. The work contains many magic remedies and incantations, and the calibre of this collection of popular prescriptions and folk remedies is not high.

Early in the fourth century A.D., an unknown compiler collected the medical passages from Pliny's *Historia naturalis* into what is variably called the *Medicina Plinii Secundi* or *Plinii valeriani*. Its compiler begins with the statement that it is written for the protection of travelers against the quackery of worthless drugs sold at high prices by avaricious physicians. Arranged in three books, the usual head-to-foot sequence is observed, and a wide choice of drugs is recommended for each ailment, with an exceptionally full discussion of antidotes against various poisons. Because of Pliny's fame, perhaps, the book was both popular and influential.

Although most of the surviving work of Soranus of Ephesus, a first or second century A.D. Greek physician, deals with gynecology, this leader of the Methodist sect of physicians was a prolific writer, and had a reputation in ancient times second only to those of Hippocrates and Galen.[38] Abridgments of his works were one of the chief means whereby the tradition of Greco-Roman medicine passed to the middle ages. Caelius Aurelianus[39] was his chief translator: about all that is known of him is that he was probably a fifth-century North African. Caelius' *De morbis acutis* and *De morbis chronicis* seem to have been based on Soranus' *Peri oxeôn kai chroniôn pathôn* and survive in incomplete form whilst the Greek original, if Caelius' works are mere translations, is lost. The discussion of each disease in Caelius usually begins with an etymology and includes a systematic discussion of differential diagnosis, therapy, and very often full reviews of dissenting opinions. There is a vague reference to what may be this writer in Cassiodorus,[40]

and certain of the *Medicinales responsiones* attributed to Caelius are listed in catalogues of monastery libraries at Lorsch, Reichenau, and St. Gallen during the ninth century. Isidore of Seville and other medieval glossarists often use language quite similar to that of Caelius or other Methodist physicians in their medical passages, but this surely reflects their manuscript sources rather than any matured, deliberate preference for the Methodist sect of physicians itself. The conclusion that a glossarist preferred one medical sect over another is usually unwarranted: he used the manuscripts before him.

The problem of the *Medicinalium responsium libri* of Caelius Aurelius is a confused one: Valentine Rose[41] conjectures that this work is a digest of Caelius Aurelianus, possibly prepared by himself, which fortuitously survived in only one manuscript, in question-and-answer form, but this seems tenuous. In 1870 Rose published the Latin texts of four medical writings which reflect very much the same spirit as the medical portions of Isidore: *Soranus de digestionibus* is a dietetic and medical work in the form of a catechism which retains some of the phrasing of Caelius Aurelianus;[42] the *Sorani Ephesii in artem medendi isagoge* Rose thinks descended from the Pseudo-Galenic *Horoi*,[43] themselves probably the remains of a second century A.D. Greek work compiled from earlier writers, of whom Rose singles out Athenaeus Attalensis (*fl. ca.* A.D. 41–54).[44] There are also two versions of a fragment on the pulse, *Soranus peri sfigmon*, which is probably a translation of an earlier work also ultimately derived from the Greek. Through all the Middle Ages, the name of Soranus is often associated with Hippocrates and Galen in reputation, but the textual relationship between the various Pseudo-Galens, Caelius Aurelius, Caelius Aurelianus and Pseudo-Soranus writings, to say nothing of their various offshoots, as they now survive is, at best, confused.

Sextus Placitus Papyriensis was a writer, probably of the fourth century, whose *De medicamentis ex*

---

[38] Sigerist believes that Caelius Aurelianus also translated Soranus' *Gynaecia* (*op. cit.*, p. 134), which was later independently made into an illustrated manual or catechism for midwives. There is a scholarly English translation by Owsei Temkin, *Soranus' Gynecology* (Baltimore, 1954), and see also M. F. Drabkin and I. E. Drabkin, *Caelius Aurelianus Gynaecia* (Baltimore, 1951).

[39] Without being able to adduce much proof, one is entitled to believe that Caelius Aurelianus was considerably more than a mere translator: arguments that he did nothing more than translate certain lost works of Soranus, like many textual and critical arguments based upon "lost" or hypothetical sources, really beg the question.

[40] Cassiodorus, *Institutiones* 1. 21. (Ed. Mynors, p. 79).

[41] The Soranus *Responsiones medicinales* are in Valentine Rose, *Anecdota graeca et graecolatina* (Berlin, 1870) 2: pp. 161–240, with the introductory material at pp. 161–180 for the Pseudo-Soranus, *Quaestiones medicinales*, the text following at pp. 241–280. "Aurelius," to which there may be a reference in Cassiodorus (see note 61, below), is published by Charles Daremberg, "Liber Aurelii de acutis passionibus," *Janus* 2 (1847): 468–499, 690–731.

[42] Codex Coll. Sloane 1122, twelfth century, collated by Rose in 1864 has the same mistakes and lacunae as a manuscript collated by him at Carlsrhue and originally in the monastery at Reichenau, which a later hand had tried to emend. The same text, untitled and with only one major lacuna, is in Codex Augiensis 120, of the ninth or tenth century.

[43] The *Horoi* are in Kühn's edition of Galen, vol. 19, pp. 348 ff. For a Latin version, see L. C. MacKinney, "Hippocratic Ethics," *Bulletin of the History of Medicine* 26 (1952): 1.

[44] A Latin text is found in a London manuscript (Codex Cotton, Galba E. IV) of the thirteenth century where it breaks off in the middle of the surgical part, leaving the text incomplete.

animalibus pecoribus et bestiis vel avibus, "Concerning medicaments derived from domestic animals and beasts or birds," survives in two differing recensions, dating to the early fifth century and does not differ from other works of this kind. Vindicianus Afer (*fl.* late fourth century) was private physician to the Emperor Valentinian I, and was converted to the Christian religion by his friend and patient, Augustine of Hippo.[45] Most of his writings have perished, but his influence survived in the works of his famous pupil, Theodore Priscian (*fl.* early fifth century), who wrote the *Euphorista* ("Cheap remedies") in Greek, from which a Latin translation was soon made. This seems to have had much in common with the Pseudo-Galenic *Peri euporistôn.* Portions dealing with definitions and diagnosis generally follow the Methodist school, and the gynecological discussions seem based on Soranus of Ephesus, suggesting eclectic origin.

Cassius Felix, another North African, compiled in A.D. 447, a short Latin epitome of the teachings of the Dogmatic school, entitled *De medicina ex Graecis logicae sectae auctoribus liber translatus.* Galen, especially the *Therapeia ad Glauconem* and the Pseudo-Galenic *Euporistôn,* contribute heavily. Cassius' work proceeds systematically, and although brief, is reasonable in its therapeutic recommendations. More attention is given to pharmaceutic and less to dietetic treatment by Dogmatic than by Methodist physicians (as represented, for example, by Caelius Aurelianus), and Cassius begins each chapter with a definition of the disease, sometimes providing an etymology. Cassius seems to have been well enough known in the early Middle Ages, but to have been overlooked from that time until Rose's *editio princeps.* Isidore's language is sometimes verbatim that of Cassius Felix.

Marcellus Empiricus (*or* Burdigalensis) of Bordeaux was Master of Offices under Theodosius I and a medical amateur still alive in 408. His *De medicamentis liber* is based on the *Medicina Plinii,* the herbal of Pseudo-Apuleius and Scribonius Largus, among others, mixed with generous quantities of folk-medicine. Apparently intended for the indigent sick, it offers nothing more than the usual ancient home remedies.

Veterinary medicine was not neglected by the ancients: Pelagonius compiled his *Veterinaria* between 363 and 366, chiefly from Greek sources, but apparently also with some reference to the agricultural writings of Celsus and Columella. Less superstitious than many of the works of the time on human medicine, it was a source for Publius (or Flavius) Vegetius Renatus, whose reputation was made by a textbook of military science, the *Epitome rei militaris,* but who

also wrote the *Digestorum artis mulomedicinae libri,* a treatise on the diseases of the mule, a work sometimes referred to as the *Ars veterinaria.*

MEDICAL GLOSS COLLECTIONS

Because of its role in general education, many individuals who never intended to practice studied medicine early in the Middle Ages, and most of this study involved reading the standard introductory medical textbooks, commentaries, and manuals found in the library. The technical medical vocabulary would prove difficult at first, and a glossary of medical terms with simple definitions would prove useful. Isidore's brief scientific and medical notes could fill such a need, and possibly he included medicine in the *Etymologiae* for this reason. A *gloss* is essentially a marginal or interlinear notation explaining a difficult word, the *lemma* word. A *scholion* is a more extensive comment, and anyone who has studied a language not native to him has been, to an extent, both glossarist and scholiast as he entered notes on the pages of his text. The next logical step is a *glossary,* or collection of glosses, wherein unfamiliar words are defined and sometimes provided with brief quotations to illustrate correct usage. In time, special authors, dialects and subjects came to have special gloss collections, and the compilation of glossaries has its basis in the study of writings which differ from ordinary speech, whether this is due to specialized subject matter or literary archaism.

Surviving Latin gloss collections date, in their present form, from about the sixth century A.D., and are customarily named from their opening word (e.g., *Glossarium ABAVUS*) or principal manuscript (e.g., *Glossarium ST. GALL*). Such collections stemmed from the practical needs of scholars who began to collect and organize marginalia from the works which passed through their hands. Amplification to any extent seems, at first, to have been infrequent, but became commoner with time, and such collections (with which much of Isidore's *Etymologiae* must be grouped) remain valuable for the interpretation of such Latin literature as, from its technical or non-literary character, is far removed from the style of the standard school authors. They help, especially, to bridge the gap between the Latin and Romance languages, often illuminate the texts of ancient writers and frequently transmit or preserve morsels of knowledge not elsewhere found. Bilingual glossaries as such seem to have made relatively a late appearance. The sixth-century *Cyrillus* glossary (Greek to Latin), the roughly contemporaneous *Philoxenus* (Latin to Greek), the *Hermeneumata* (Greek to Latin) and assorted glossaries with Latin to Anglo-Saxon, Celtic, Germanic, and other interpretations are known, and many manuscripts survive from the early Middle Ages with interlinear translations which are sometimes more than mere cribs.

---

[45] A few fragments are published by Valentine Rose as an appendix to his edition of Theodore Priscian (Leipzig, 1894), pp. 428–466, and Wellmann published fragments in *Fragmentensammlung der griechischen Ärzte* 1 (1901): 208–234. On his relations with Augustine, see *Confessions* 4. 3. 5; 7. 6. 8 and Augustine, *Epistola* 138. 3.

The arrangement of the words in medical gloss collections [46] was alphabetical by first letters or, about as frequently, topical in the head-to-foot sequence used in Egypt and retained, for example, in Rufus of Ephesus' (fl. ca. A.D. 98–117) Greek *On the names of the parts of the human body*, where he discusses the anatomical names of bodily organs and sometimes provides etymologies of very considerable length. This philological interest had developed slowly: the Hippocratic school had little of it and it is not marked in Galen, but is well developed in Soranus, Cassius Felix, and Caelius Aurelianus. Isidore generally follows the head-to-foot arrangement in his books on medicine and anatomy. Alphabetical arrangement by the first letter or, more rarely, by the first two letters was less frequent during the early Middle Ages for medical works, but was often followed in handbooks of therapeutics and materia medica, and was the rule for medical glossaries, lexica and concordances.

In these glossaries, difficult and unfamiliar or technical words are defined in more familiar terms, of which W. M. Lindsay remarks:

We need have no suspicion of the Latin used to explain difficult words to monastery students. We may be sure that the explanations written first in the margins of texts, and transferred from there to a list of *glossae collectae* and ultimately to a monastery dictionary, a *glossarium* or *liber glossarum*, were real explanations; they would be couched in the most familiar, the most natural, language, the language most intelligible to the monastery students for whose benefit they were written.[47]

A common feature of glossaries, obvious in Isidore's definitions, is the *id est* formula: the *lemma*, or word to be defined, is stated in the nominative case, followed by *id est* (= "that is") and a definition which might be a single word, or a long discussion including not only an etymology but a conspectus of authoritative opinions and examples of correct use. When Greek words were first contributing to a Latin medical vocabulary, demand arose for Greek-to-Latin glossaries, none of which seem to have survived in their original form. These may have been compiled from strictly medical sources but seem more often to have been excerpted from general gloss collections. Isidore's *Etymologiae* IV deals with medicine, and his definitions—many of them extremely brief and fragmentary—suggest that they have been taken from medical texts essentially written by and for physicians. The generally fuller definitions of anatomic terms found in *Etymologiae* XI contain less technical material, suggesting that the anatomic terms were derived from general literary sources, including the encyclopedias and commentaries on standard writers current in Isidore's time.

Referring to the seven volumes of Keil's *Grammatici latini*,[48] containing so many of the philological writings of postclassical times, Henry Nettleship notes that they

... appear to contain a large number of independent grammatical treatises, which bear different names, and are often quoted as the works of independent authors. A nearer study of them soon reveals the fact that they consist, in large part, of matter nearly or quite identical; that the same rules, lists, and instances served as the stock in trade of a great number of different professors at various times and in distant places; and that the whole mass might probably be so sifted as to reduce the bulk of original work to a comparatively small amount, and enable us to refer it to the authorship of probably less than a dozen scholars, none of them later than the age of the Antonines.[49]

MEDICINE AND THE WESTERN FATHERS

The fathers of the Western Church included medicine in their general educational programs, but an informed interest in medicine is not the practice of medicine. The structure and function of the human body are used by Churchmen to illustrate the wisdom and goodness of God, and their study is not always subordinated to ethical views or to the exigencies of explaining the world of sensible creation. Their concern with medical and scientific subjects not only imparted a certain intellectual respectability, but ensured medicine a place in Church-dominated educational programs. A wholly new attitude toward the care of the sick and unfortunate was inculcated, which improved the general reputation of medicine even as an intellectual discipline.

The medical views of early Churchmen reflect a correctly understood but highly oversimplified Galenic physiology with its later localization of the emotions: joy in the spleen, carnal love in the liver, knowledge in the heart and anger in the bile. Occasionally, specific diseases are mentioned in theological or moral contexts, but usually without very exact descriptions. The threat of mental or physical illness as a punishment for a specific sin is rare: disease is thought to stem from natural causes and the resources of human medicine must be invoked, although God may permit man to fall sick and to suffer for His own inscrutable ends.

---

[46] W. M. Lindsay, "The Editing of Isidore, *Etymologiae*," *The Classical Quarterly* 5 (1911): 42, notes that both the *Glossarium Ansileubus* and the *Lexicon* of Julian of Toledo (ob. 690) borrow from Isidore. For an account of Isidore's influence on Anglo-Saxon glossariography, see R. T. Meyer, "Isidorian 'Glossae Collectae' in Aelfric's vocabulary," *Traditio* 12 (1956): 398. On medical gloss collections in general, see L. C. MacKinney, "Medieval Medical Dictionaries and Glossaries," *Medieval and Historiographical Studies in Honor of James Westfall Thompson* (Chicago, 1938); P. Jourdan, "A Propos des 'glossae medicinales,'" *Bulletin du Cange* 3 (1927): 121, who has some comments on Rose's text of *Aurelius de passionibus;* and A. Thomas, "Notes lexicographiques sur recettes médicales du haut moyen age," *Bulletin du Cange* 5 (1930): 97.

[47] W. M. Lindsay, "Note on the Use of Glossaries for the Dictionary of Medieval Latin," *Bulletin du Cange* 1 (1924): 16.

[48] H. Keil, ed., *Grammatici latini* (7 v., Leipzig, 1857–1880).

[49] Henry Nettleship, *Lectures and Essays: Second Series* (Oxford, 1895), p. 145.

In the subapostolic age, Clement of Alexandria's (*ca.* 150–211) detailed exposition of the moral teachings of Christ, the *Paedagogus,* and his discusion of the superiority of Christian to Greek philosophy, the *Stromateis,* outline a strongly teleological psychology based on Greek sources. His great influence in the West was through Latin translations which appeared soon after these works were composed. The erudite but erratic Tertullian (*ca.* 160–*ca.* 225), a North African lawyer, although no physician, was widely read in Greek and Latin scientific literature, and was familiar with some of Galen and the scientific portions of Plato and Aristotle. He refers to a lost work of Soranus of Ephesus on philosophical psychology, the *De anima,* which seems to reflect the doctrine of Plato, Aristotle, Chrysippus, and Heraclides of Pontus. In discussing the surgical instruments used in fetal craniotomy, an operation abhorrent to Christian morals, Tertullian refers to Soranus as "kindly"—*mitior ipse Soranus* [50]—suggesting that he knew his medical works, valuable sources not only for Greco-Roman medicine, but for their etymologies.[51] Tertullian leans toward the Methodist sect, although this may reflect only the sources available to him, and in his own *De anima,* a well-documented and closely reasoned work, he attempts to synthesize classical scientific and Christian philosophical thought. Despite his subsequent lapse into heresy, he is the first important Christian Latin writer.

A calmer writer than Tertullian was Caecilius Firmianus Lactantius (*ca.* 250–*ca.* 317), a pupil of Arnobius, who wrote in Asia Minor during the last of Diocletian's persecutions "On the workmanship of God"—*De opificio Dei.* Based entirely on other writings, this work interprets the structure and function of the human body to demonstrate Divine goodness: brief, enthusiastic, and extremely clear, it was an indispensable work all through the early Christian era. Augustine, Bishop of Hippo (354–430), by far the most influential Christian thinker between Paul and Luther, formulated in his numerous writings—about six times in bulk those which survive of Cicero—a firmly realist Christian psychology and epistemology. He does not undertake to write on medicine or physiology, as such, but his writings frequently touch upon such matters. He

mentions the three cerebral ventricles known to ancient anatomists, in the walls (or on the meninges) of which were thought to reside anteriorly, sensation, centrally memory and posteriorly thought.[52] He mentions respiration,[53] and in his discussion of the gastrointestinal tract, distinguishes between the stomach's digestion of food and the intestine's transportation and elimination.[54] His teleology is complete,[55] and by way of parenthesis, his condemnation of abortion [56] as equivalent to murder and stand against contraception [57] remain conservative Christian moral principles.

Ambrose (*ca.* 337–397), though less erudite than Tertullian or Augustine, in his commentary on the Genesis account of creation, the *Hexameron,* likewise reflects the physiological notions current in his day. He mentions, for example, that the pulse is an index of health and disease,[58] and repeats the venerable Pythagorean teaching that semen is derived from the kidneys and spinal cord.[59] The liver digests food into vapor, and the brain is the seat of sensation and the center of all nerves, so that Ambrose disagrees with those who located thought and sensation in the heart.[60] Neither Ambrose nor Augustine wrote separate scientific works, as did Tertullian and Lactantius, but they mentioned these topics during theological and moral discussions, apparently confident that cultivated nonmedical people would be familiar with them.

Cassiodorus had urged the copying and study of medical works, and provided for medical studies in his *Institutes.* Although familiar, his observations bear quotation:

On Doctors. I salute you, distinguished brothers, who with sedulous care look after the health of the human body and perform the functions of blessed piety for those who flee to the shrines of holy men—you who are sad at the sufferings of others, sorrowful for those who are in danger, grieved at the pain of those who are received, and always distressed with personal sorrow at the misfortunes of others, so that, as experience of your art teaches, you help the sick with genuine zeal; you will receive your reward from Him by Whom eternal rewards may be paid for temporal acts. Learn, therefore, the properties of herbs and perform the compounding of drugs punctiliously; but do not place your hope in herbs and do not trust health to human counsels. For although the art of medicine be found to be established by the Lord, He Who without doubt grants life to men makes them sound. For it is written: "And whatsoever ye do in word or deed, do all in the name of the Lord Jesus, giving thanks to God and the Father by Him."

But if the eloquence of Greek letters is unknown to you, you have first of all the *Herb Book* of Dioscorides, who has treated and portrayed the herbs of the fields with remarkable accuracy. After this read the Latin translation of

[50] Tertullian, *De anima* 25. 5.

[51] E. A. Quain, *Tertullian, Apologetical Works and Minucius Felix, Octavius* (New York, 1950), p. 191, in a note on Tertullian, *De anima* 6. 6, comments without stating his sources: "Soranus, a Greek physician of the early second century A.D., wrote four books on the soul, in which he quoted from the works of Plato, Aristotle, Chrysippus, and Heraclides of Pontus. He was keenly interested in the history of medicine and etymology. Much of Tertullian's information about medical matters and ancient Greek religion is apparently borrowed from Soranus."

For an attempted reconstruction of Soranus's work on the soul, see Heinrich Karpp, "Sorans vier Bücher Περὶ ψυχῆς und Tertullians Schrift De Anima," *Zeitschrift für die Neutestamentliche Wissenschaft und die Kunde der Älterenkirche* 33 (1934) : 31–47.

[52] Augustine, *De Genesi ad litteram* 7. 18 [*PL* 34: 364]
[53] Augustine, *De anima* 2. 4 [*PL* 44: 573].
[54] Augustine, *Sermo* 243. 6–7 [*PL* 38: 1146].
[55] Augustine, *Sermo* 24. 5 [*PL* 38: 165].
[56] Augustine, *De nuptiis et concupiscentia* 2. 12 [*PL* 44: 450].
[57] Genesis 38: 8–10.
[58] Ambrose, *Hexameron* 6. 9 [*PL* 14: 264].
[59] *Ibid.* [*PL* 14: 271], see Isidore, XI. 1. 104 below.
[60] *Ibid.* [*PL* 14: 268].

Hippocrates and Galen [That is, the *Therapeutics* of Galen, addressed to the philosopher Glauco] and a certain anonymous work, which has been compiled from various authors. Finally, read Caelius Aurelius' *On medicine*, and Hippocrates *On herbs and cures*, and various other works written on the art of medicine; with God's help, I have left you these books, stored away in the recesses of our library.[61]

The Church, during this period, did not limit its concern with medicine to an occasional sermon comment. Benedict of Nursia ordered that the sick be carefully attended in the monasteries following his rule and earlier, Basil of Cappadocia, said to have had "some" knowledge of medicine, made similar provisions. By the sixth century, the study of compendia of classical medicine was an established part of monastic routine, and the monks themselves provided simple nursing care for those living in their houses. A monastery included a large variety as well as number of people: its abbot (whom Benedict envisioned exactly as a Roman *paterfamilias*), monks, lay brothers, students of varying ages, permanent and transient guests, serfs ascribed to monastery lands, hired servants, their families and those hangers-on found in all institutions in every age, together with many of the sick, aged, and destitute of the neighborhood who depended upon charity to keep body and soul together.

Some were ill to begin with and others became so: Benedict, as usual, is direct, explicit and practical:

Of the Sick Brethren. Before all things and above all things care is to be had of the sick, that they be served in very deed as Christ Himself, for He hath said: "I was sick, and ye visited Me." And, "What ye have done unto one of these little ones, ye have done unto Me." And let the sick themselves remember that they are served for the honour of God, and not grieve the brethren who serve them by unnecessary demands. Yet must they be patiently borne with, because from such as these is gained a more abundant reward. Let it be, therefore, the Abbot's greatest care that they suffer no neglect. And let a cell be set apart by itself for the sick brethren, and one who is God-fearing, diligent and careful, be appointed to serve them. Let the use of baths be allowed to the sick as often as may be expedient; but to those who are well, and especially to the young, let it be granted more seldom. Let the use of flesh meat also be permitted to the sick and to those who are very weakly, for their recovery: but when they are restored to health, let all abstain from meat in the accustomed manner. The Abbot must take all possible care that the sick be not neglected by the Cellarer or servers; because whatever is done amiss by his disciples is laid to his charge.[62]

Care of the monastery sick seems to have been intelligent and humane. Most monasteries had herb gardens and monks skilled in their use, who carried on for centuries the herbal prescriptions of classical antiquity. If most of these herbs did little good, they did little harm, and many patients may wisely have preferred prayer to the more heroic therapy available. Minor surgical procedures, including seasonal bloodletting, were undertaken, but extensive surgical operations were rare inside or outside monasteries.

The practice of medicine no less than other social institutions changed as western Europe recovered from the chaos which followed the Roman collapse. Medical practice by laymen had always existed: a capitular of Charlemagne in 805 provided that everyone learn some mathematics at school, and that some young men be sent to study medicine. Likely these would, just as in postclassical times, pass some years with an established physician of good reputation, study the standard medical texts, and visit patients with him, since both clerical and lay physicians continued both to practice and to teach apprentices.[63] Later, the Council of Tours forbade regular (i.e., monastic as opposed to parish) clergy to attend law and, possibly, medical schools. Although limited to one jurisdiction, this suggests that Church authorities were uneasy about clerical medical practice.[64] As lay practitioners increased in number,

[61] Cassiodorus, *Institutiones* 1. 21 [Mynors, 78–79] translation: L. W. Jones, *An introduction to divine and human readings by Cassiodorus Senator* [New York, 1946], pp. 135–136. Sigerist (*op. cit.*, p. 133) notes: "What Cassiodorus meant under *Hippocratis de herbis* is hard to tell. No such book occurs in the Corpus Hippocraticum. What is meant is perhaps the so-called *Dynamidia Hippocratis* which is based on the Hippocratic treatise *De diaeta*, Book III, and includes excerpts from Gargilius Martialis."

G. R. J. Fletcher, "St. Isidore of Seville and his book on medicine" *Proceedings of the Royal Society of Medicine* 12 (1919): 76–77, comments: "*Reconditos* suggests MSS on special subjects stored away as not for general reading. An interesting question arises, whether 'Aurelius Coelius' is Aurelius Celsus or Coelius Aurelianus. The title of the work of Celsus is *De Medicina*, and no work of Aurelianus is known under that designation. At Vivarium therefore in the sixth century there was a fair collection of books on medicine by both Greek and Latin authors. Isidore had an extensive library of general literature and, as we shall see presently, one of the chests was reserved for works on medical subjects."

At p. 90: "In 1847 Daremberg had published a MS, preserved at Brussels, entitled 'Aurelius *de Morbis Acutis*' which on examination was found to be an epitome of the *De Morbis Acutis* of Aurelianus, and some observations on fever (possibly part of the lost work of Aurelianus)."

The evidence suggests that Cassiodorus refers to a work similar to, but not necessarily identical to, the Daremberg text. Fletcher is certainly correct when he states that certain books were set aside in monastery libraries for those with special interests, including medicine. *Depinxit* in the citation from Cassiodorus refers to the illustrated herbals in use through the early middle ages, but Fletcher is surely incorrect in suggesting that Cornelius Celsus is the medical writer intended. Valentine Rose [*Hermes* 8 (1874): 38] suggests the herbal mentioned by Cassiodorus is Pseudo-Dioscorides. The Hippocratic *De herbis et curis* was probably one of many pseudonymous late Latin medical compilations.

[62] Oswald Hunter-Blair, *The Rule of St. Benedict* (5th ed., Fort Augustus, 1948), pp. 100–103, Chapter 36, "De infirmis fratribus."

[63] Léon Maitre, *Les Écoles épiscopales et monastiques en occident avant les universites* (2nd ed., Paris, 1924), p. 11, quotes: *De computo ut veraciter discant omnes; de medicina arte, ut infantes hanc discere mittantur.*

[64] Johannes Maan, *Turonensis provinciae concilia*, p. 90, quoted by Maitre, *op. cit.*, p. 165: *Ne regulares e claustris exeant seculares adituri scholas ad legendas leges et confectiones physicas ponderandas.* This *confectiones physicas ponderandas*

Church officials seem to have preferred that priests and monks withdraw from practice: the problem does not seem to have been the spirit of fornication but that of avarice.

ISIDORE'S *DE NATURA RERUM* AND *ETYMOLOGIAE*

Isidore was a prolific, if unoriginal, writer, and not all of his works have survived. Those which have may be generally classified as:

I. Compilations: (*a*) The *Etymologiae*, an encyclopedic dictionary; (*b*) *Libri duo differentiarum* and *De differentiis verborum*, discussions of the differences between words apparently synonymous; (*c*) *De differentiis rerum*, a theological glossary; (*d*) *De natura rerum*, a treatise on cosmology; as is also (*e*) *De ordine creaturarum*.

II. Historical works: (*a*) The *Chronica*, extending to A.D. 615, based primarily upon Julius Africanus, Eusebius, Jerome and Victor of Tunnuna, although certain manuscripts have been continued to A.D. 627; (*b*) The *Historia de regibus Gothorum, Vandalorum et Suevorum*, a regional history demonstrating Isidore's consciousness of himself as a Spaniard; and (*c*) *De viris illustribus*, essentially a catalogue of Christian writers, a continuation of Jerome and Gennadius.

III. Scriptural Commentary: Isidore's approach is historical rather than exegetical. (*a*) *De ortu et obitu patrum qui in scriptura laudibus efferuntur*, a history of the patriarchs and saints of the Old and New Testaments; (*b*) *Allegoriae quaedam sacrae scripturae*, an allegorical interpretation of certain passages from Holy Scripture; (*c*) *Liber numerorum qui in sanctis scripturis occurrunt*, a mystical interpretation of the numbers mentioned in scripture; (*d*) *In libros veteris et novi testamenti prooemia*, brief introductions to the books of the Old and New Testaments; (*e*) *De veteri et novo testamento quaestiones*, a collection of set solutions to certain problems in exegesis; and (*f*) *Mysticorum expositiones sacramentorum seu quaestiones in vetus testamentum*, allegorical interpretations of certain Old Testament events.

IV. Theological works: (*a*) *De fide catholica ex veteri et novo testamento contra Iudaeos ad Florentinam sororem suam*, an apologetic for Christianity against the Jews, and (*b*) *Libri tres sententiarum*, a selection largely from the writings of Gregory the Great which amounts to a manual of moral and dogmatic theology.

V. Liturgiology: The *De ecclesiasticis officiis*, "On the duties of Churchmen," deals with the different parts of divine worship and with the sacraments of the Church, and with the relationships and duties of the clergy and layfolk of the Church.

Miscellaneous works include ascetical writings and some correspondence: his *Regula monachorum* seems to have been independent of that of Benedict, and to have been little used in practice. Isidore gave much attention to canon law and ceremonial matters, and although a number of hymns and letters have been attributed to him, most of these are considered spurious.

At some time before 620, Isidore began to compile an encyclopedia which was probably related to his plans for higher education in his diocese, and parts of the encyclopedia were circulated during that year.[65] The work was dedicated to King Sisebut, who died in July, 620. It is likely that Isidore made very extensive notes, with considerable secretarial help, on his reading over many years, grouping these by subject matter, and that as the years passed, these accumulated.[66] Gradually, this material was sifted and new divisions were added. Although the first books dealt with the liberal arts and were probably based, like so many textbooks, on the curriculum at Isidore's cathedral school, where Isidore may have himself taught, there were many miscellaneous topics which had to be arranged by Braulio, even after the earlier publication of portions of *Etymologiae* I–VIII most useful to students of the liberal arts.[67]

Since Isidore did not live to complete a final revision, the present Latin text of the *Etymologiae* depends in large part on Braulio's editing: Braulio had spent ten years or so as Isidore's student and associate before he became Bishop of Saragossa, and their correspondence affecting the *Etymologiae* is printed as a preface to most of the texts. The *Etymologiae* form a very long work —two thick volumes in the Oxford Classical series— and a single scribe would have needed something like a year to make a copy of it in the unadorned book-hand of the period. The manuscript which Isidore, an old and ailing man, sent Braulio seems to have been the *codex inemendatus* mentioned in a letter which Lynch dates at 632,[68] and to have contained many blemishes, omis-

[65] Isidore's own view of the *Etymologiae* is summarized in Epistola VI (Isidore to Sisebut), about 632: "I am sending you, as I promised that I would, a work concerning the origin of certain things collected from notes by older writers and annotated in certain places, so that it stands as though written by the pen of our elders."

[66] A card-catalogue, or scissors-and-paste, origin for the *Etymologiae* is suggested by such frequent repetitions as: X. 129, †tur† *enim flamma dicitur*, which the editors amend to πῦρ; II. 12. 6, *ignis enim apud Graecos* πῦρ *appellatur;* XV. 11. 4, πῦρ *enim dicitur ignis;* and XVI. 1, 9, πῦρ *enim ignis est.*

[67] Lynch, *op. cit.,* pp. 42–44.

[68] Epistola V (Isidore to Braulio): "Your reverence's letters reached me in the city of Toledo, where I had gone to attend the council. . . . While on the journey, I sent you the codex of the *Etymologies,* along with some other books, and, although uncorrected because of my illness, still I desired to send them to you at least for correction, if I should have arrived at the place appointed for the council."

Lynch, *op. cit.,* pp. 33–54, discusses the letters between

is a strange circumlocution: *ars medendi* or merely *medicina* or *re medica* would have been more to the point, and more idiomatic. This may refer to the preparation of prescriptions, which possibly involved alchemy, the confection of love philters, providing poisons and other questionable activity.

sions, lacunae, mistaken citations, repetitions, and bald errors. Whether these were due to Isidore, his secretaries, his sources or his scribes is unimportant: the sources he used may have been corrupt, and possibly there were passages whose precise meaning was unknown to Isidore himself.[69] Isidore appointed Braulio his literary executor, and the traditional division of the *Etymologiae* into twenty books was made by him. Braulio's *Praenotatio*,[70] which Lynch dates at 637,[71] notes that Isidore wrote the *Etymologiae* at his request, but that he edited it in its final form.

The *Etymologiae* is a dictionary of the liberal arts, much like those of Martianus Capella and Cassiodorus, and an encyclopedia after the manner of Varro and Verrius Flaccus in literary and antiquarian scope, and Pliny in scientific matters. Like any compilation, it is dry and disconnected reading, and Isidore rarely permits himself spontaneity: his encomium on the noble character of the dog is almost an isolated exception.[72] He does not overlook certain subjects which might offend certain readers' feelings of propriety, and foresaw this criticism.[73] There are many errors in the *Etymologiae*, but there is little magic in the medical and scientific parts. Later, Rhabanus Maurus (776–856) based his own encyclopedia, the *De sermonum proprietate*, on Isidore's work, and adopted the medical portions almost *in toto*. Rhabanus mixed more religion with his medicine than did Isidore and, to that extent, is less objective. The medical portions of Rhabanus' encyclopedia, derived from Isidore, are sometimes considered the first medical work printed from type during the Renaissance.[74]

For Isidore, as for most of those concerned with learning during the patristic age, it was from the classical tradition, rethought in the light of Christian faith and morals, that useful knowledge would come. Preoccupation with origins, with basic causes, characterizes Isidore's work, and he accords such origins more attention in his analyses and analogies than he does the elemental theory so widely accepted by the men of his time. For Isidore, words and letters are in a sense elements into which spoken and written words can be reduced, and from which careful analysis will derive valuable insights and understanding. Sarton notes:

[the] importance generally attached to names and words, whether it be under the influence of philosophy or religion or magic, increased enormously the interest in philological studies.[75]

At the beginning of the *Differentiarum*, Isidore recalled that many ancient attempts had been made to explain the often subtle differences between words, and he consistently assumes that the way to knowledge is through words in terms of their origins rather than in terms of their logical meanings. He undertook to clarify word-meanings with regard to origins amid a confusion of false usage so that they could find their own proper place in the fabric of truth. So thoroughly was Isidore a Platonist that, for him, words are all but transcendentals.

Henry Osborne Taylor remarks, of the *Etymologiae*, "The dryness of this work and its poverty of thought are outdone only by the absurdity of its etymologies," [76] and Brehaut adds, "He tells us practically nothing concerning his own period in which so many important changes were taking place." [77] Thorndike, however, observes:

Isidore seems . . . to display a notable power of brief generalization, of terse expression and telling use of words. We should not have to go back to the middle ages for textbook writers who have written more and said less. This power of condensed expression probably accounts for Isidore's being so much cited.[78]

Floyd Seyward Lear's 1936 lecture on Isidore concludes:

Isidore and Braulio concerning the *Etymologiae*. Braulio seems to have been Isidore's closest friend for, in Epistola III, Isidore thanks him for the gift of a parrot which he kept in a cage in his room.

[69] Isidore followed no one system of orthography and no one method in his compilations, nor does he always provide the same derivation for a word (see XVI. 21. 3 and XIX. 10. 1, for example) and he sometimes (e.g., IV.7.36) seems to use a variant spelling for the sake of his etymology. Isidore's orthography reflects variation in spelling among his sources no less than the changes which were taking place in the Latin language. There are some variant readings (e.g., IV. 7. 6) best explicable if the archetypal manuscript had variant readings.

[70] S. *Braulionis Caesaraugustani episcopi praenotatio librorum D. Isidori* [*PL* 81: 15–17, 82: 65–68].

[71] Lynch, *op. cit.*, p. 212.

[72] XII. 2. 25–26.

[73] Epistola IV, *ad finem*: ". . . Nor shall I pass over in silence those things which I sought for and found. But you leave a way open for the hope that, on the face of it, you will not pierce me with the goads of my shame and worthlessness, and that you cherish whatever you find that does not deserve to be denounced. . . ."

[74] E. C. Jessup, "Rabanus Maurus: 'De sermonum proprietate, seu de universo,'" *Annals of Medical History*, n. s., 6 (1934): 35, gives an English translation of Rhabanus' book 18, chapter 5, "On Medicine and Diseases," although he does not mention Isidore or his medical writings as sources. An edition of Rhabanus Maurus, *De universo* (Strasburg, 1467) antedates

the *editio princeps* of Isidore's *Etymologiae* by three years. (Medieval manuscript catalogues refer to Rhabanus' works as *Liber etymologiarum* or *De naturis rerum*: "*De universo*" is a modern title.) E. K. Graham, *The de universo of Hrabanus Maurus: a mediaeval encyclopedia* (Typescript M.A. thesis, University of North Carolina, 1934) gives a satisfactory account of Rhabanus' use of Isidore's *Etymologiae*.

[75] George Sarton, *Introduction to the History of Science* (Washington, 1927) 1: 23.

[76] H. O. Taylor, *The Mediaeval Mind* (4th ed., Cambridge, Mass., 1949) 1: p. 51.

[77] Brehaut, *op. cit.*, p. 33, and see Theodor Mommsen, ed., *Isidori . . . Chronica* in the *Monumenta germaniae historica* (Berlin, 1894).

[78] Lynn Thorndike, *A History of Magic and Experimental Science during the First Thirteen Centuries of Our Era* (London, 1929) 1: pp. 624–625.

... he was one of those towering figures, conspicuous in mediaeval times, whose names lent prestige to various works by virtue of false attribution. Isidore's pseudonymousness ranges from the famous *False Decretals* in canon law to various minor lyric poems. And W. P. Ker in his little book, *The Dark Ages*, provides a bit of final evidence in a line from the English version of the romance of the *Destruction of Troy* which he says " is as good an instance as could be found of [the saint's] popularity," at least among the half-learned—"And Ysidre in Ethemoleger openly tellis." It is a simple line; even so, dictionaries and their authors seldom figure in popular fiction.[79]

The *Etymologiae* forms a comprehensive encyclopedic dictionary. Book I deals with grammar and its various subdivisions, Book II with rhetoric and dialectic and Book III with mathematics: arithmetic, music, geometry and astronomy. Book IV deals with medicine. Book V considers laws and instruments of judgment, and units of time. Book VI discusses the order of scriptures, cycles and canons, feasts and the divine offices of worship; Book VII is concerned with God and the angels, names, names of the fathers, with martyrs, clerics, monks, and other names; and Book VIII takes up the Church and the synagogue, religion and faith, heretics, philosophers, poets, sibyls and the magi, the pagans and pagan divinities. Book IX deals with the languages of the nations, kings, and the names and relationships of civil and military affairs. Book X lists and defines certain names in roughly alphabetical order. Book XI discusses man and the parts of the human body, the ages of man, portents and transformations. Book XII takes up quadrupeds, reptiles, fish, and flying creatures; Book XIII the elements, the heavens, the air, waters, sea, rivers, and floods; and Book XIV geography, including heaven, earth, the provinces of the whole world, islands, mountains and the names of other places and the lower parts of the earth. Book XV deals with cities, urban and rural buildings, fields, boundaries and the measurement of fields and journeys, including various means of travel. Book XVI is about stones from the earth or waters, gems, common and precious stones, ivory and marble, glass, metals, weights, and measures. Book XVII is on agriculture, crops, vines, trees, fruits, vegetables, and herbs. Book XVIII discusses wars, triumphs, the instruments for waging war, the forum, games and spectacles, armor, and weapons. Book XIX is about ships, ship-chandling and rigging, metal smithing, building construction, and various things pertaining to houses, clothing, ornament, and vesture. The last Book, XX, discusses tables, food, drink, and the necessary utensils, the tools used by vinters, water and cooking, baking and lighting, beds, furniture, vehicles, country life and pleasure gardens, and saddlery.

Aside from the medical and anatomical portions, there is much in the *Etymologiae* of scientific interest: astronomy (Book III), meteorology and the elements (Book XIII), the seasons (Book V) and botany (Book

XVII). Parts of Book XII deal with zoology. Isidore's cosmological views are outlined in the *De natura rerum* and *De ordine creaturarum,* and in some respects, the *Libri differentiarum* supplement the *Etymologiae* XI, if not very usefully for the historian of science. In the *Sententiae,* the microcosm is again explained in terms of the macrocosm. *Etymologiae* XIII. 13, "On the different kinds of waters," includes a discussion of medicinal springs but like the considerations of diet and clothing in *Etymologiae* XX, lacks the scientific flavor of *Etymologiae* IV and XI.

The *De natura rerum* is a short book composed for and dedicated to Sisebut, outlining the commonly received ideas of Isidore's time on astronomy and meteorology, with a passing mention of the plague, which was thought to depend upon prevailing winds and climate. Beginning with a discussion of various divisions of time, important in view of the complex Church calendar, it proceeds to consideration of the sun, moon, planets, and stars, to end with accounts of miscellaneous natural phenomena, including the Nile, earthquakes, and Mount Etna, the only active volcano then known. His sources seem to have included Hyginus, Solinus, Ambrose's *Hexameron* (based in turn on those of Basil and Origen), Augustine of Hippo, Jerome, the Pseudo-Clementine *Recognitiones,* Suetonius, Macrobius, Aratus, Cicero, Lucretius, Pliny, Varro, Servius' Vergil Commentaries or similar material, and doubtless others, but whether at first hand or from derivative material is uncertain. The same material is presented in corresponding parts of the *Etymologiae.*

THE TEXTUAL TRADITION OF ISIDORE'S WORKS

Lindsay divides the ninth century and earlier manuscripts of the *Etymologiae* into three distinct textual families: later manuscript texts are often confused by an admixture of rival textual traditions and interpolations, no less than the errors of all manuscript tradition:

I, the "French or whole" family represents a commonly received text, and the oldest surviving manuscript was copied at Bobbio during the eighth century. Its readings are occasionally mixed with readings similar to those of

II, the "Italian or contracted" family. This may represent the text of Isidore's uncorrected archetype or, less likely, an early abridgment of a longer original. The two oldest surviving manuscripts were apparently copied from the same exemplar in the same scriptorium in Northern Italy early in the eighth century. This family represents the briefest possible text, and Lindsay suggests that its ancestor was brought from Spain to Italy no later than the end of the seventh century.

III, the "Spanish or interpolated" family, contains many interpolations and more of the *lemma* words left blank in the codices of families I and II are defined in family III than in these texts, leading Lindsay to suggest that this text is essentially Braulio's revision.

---

[79] Lear, *op. cit.,* p. 79.

If so, family II is the older text. Braulio's see city in Spain was Saragossa (*Caesaraugusta Terraconensis*),[80] a city fully described in the codices of family III but missing from those of II. Manuscripts of family III seem chiefly of Spanish origin, and the later medieval tradition of family III seems very largely independent of families I and II. The oldest surviving manuscript dates from the eighth or ninth century.

Isidore's writings generally, and the *Etymologiae* in particular, enjoyed wide popularity through the Middle Ages, and few libraries of any pretensions were without at least a volume of extracts. It is now quite impossible to say how many manuscripts of the *Etymologiae*, in part or complete, were to be found in European libraries at the dawn of the Renaissance, but some idea of their impressive distribution may be gained from Beeson's survey of manuscripts surviving in catalogued libraries which were copied before the tenth century.[81] Since these older manuscripts are the most useful in establishing a sound text, Beeson's census does not take into account eleventh-century and later manuscripts. It is perhaps fair to suggest that, so far as nonliturgical works are concerned, manuscripts of the *Etymologiae* were exceeded in number only by those of the vulgate text of the Bible.[82]

The *Etymologiae* were often reprinted during the first century after the invention of printing, usually in some variation of the commonly received text. Bermúdez Camacho and Arqués list [83] incunabula editions, fourteen of them between 1470 and 1509. The *Etymologiae* found a steady market, and the first printed editions of Isidore's complete works are those of Michael Somnius (Paris, 1580); Gomez (Madrid, 1599) and the Benedictine Du Breul (Paris, 1601, reprinted at Cologne, 1617). John Grial prepared, at the royal command, a scholarly edition of the *Etymologiae* and certain other Isidorian works (Madrid, 1599), reprinted without much change by Ulloa (Madrid, 1778), but the generally best edition of the vulgate text is that of the Jesuit Faustinus Arevalo (Rome, 1797–1803, 7 volumes), reprinted by Migne in the *Patrologia latina*, volumes 81–84. The most useful text of the *Etymologiae* is that of Wallace M. Lindsay in the *Scriptorum classicorum bibliotheca Oxoniensis* (Oxford, 1911, 2 volumes).

---

[80] XV. 1. 66.

[81] C. H. Beeson, "Isidor-Studien," *Quellen und Untersuchungen zur Lateinischen Philologie des Mittelalters* (Munich, 1913) 4: 174.

[82] See G. Becker, *Catalogi bibliothecarum antiqui* (Bonn, 1885), or P. Lehmann, *Mittelalterliche Bibliothekskataloge* (Munich, 1918), which offer catalogues of medieval libraries. Augusto Beccaria, *I codici di medicina del periodo presalernitano* (Rome, 1956) surveys early medical manuscripts, but an interesting account of some less famous but perhaps on that score more typical medieval libraries in Léon Maitre, *op. cit.*, pp. 187–203, lists Isidore's name at least once on each save four pages.

[83] *Isidorus Hispalensis Ethimologiarum liber IIII de Medicina* (Barcelona, 1945), pp. 67–68.

ISIDORE'S SOURCES

Evaluation and identification of the sources used by an ancient encyclopedist in his compilations are always uncertain, lacking citation by name at a time when neither copyright law nor scholarly convention so required. It is never safe and may be foolhardy to presume that verbal similarity between author "A" who happens to have written a generation earlier than author "B" implies that author "A" is beholden, directly or indirectly, to author "B" for his ideas or their expression, or that an influence of any kind can be predicated. There has always been a common body of scholarly and scientific information to which anyone has or can gain access, and an apparently original or prior conclusion or statement may stem from a common source long since lost, from identical or similar sources, or from parallel but independent origins. Influence may exist, but its proof is rigorous and requires much more than opportunity. This problem is complicated by the loss of many important works once popular, by the lack of scientific critical texts for many early medieval writers and by the uncertainty induced by the recollection that the accepted reading of a given text fifteen centuries ago need not have been that now taken to be correct. Few libraries, ancient or modern, are completely catalogued and fewer still of such catalogues have survived from medieval times to us, so that any opinion on the acquisition and interchange of books, whether by individuals or by institutions, rests to a large extent on fragmentary evidence and upon conjecture.

Although little direct evidence can be adduced concerning the exact literary sources, whether original works, collections of extracts or vaguely-recalled readings, for Isidore's works, various surmises have been made from his writings and quotations as to the books to which he had, at one time or another, access. Such efforts tend to err on the side of incompleteness rather than of exaggeration, and although never conclusive, do permit some definition of the *kind* (if not the precise titles and authors) of material at his disposal. Brehaut, speaking of Isidore's library, notes:

It seems probable that his working library contained works of the following authors: Lactantius, Tertullian, Jerome, Ambrose, Augustine, Orosius, Cassiodorus, Suetonius, Pliny, Solinus, Hyginus, Sallust, Hegesippus, the abridger of Vitruvius, Servius, the scholia on Lucan, and Justinus.[84]

Dressel adds Lucretius, although he probably overestimates the influence of Suetonius' lost *Prata*. Arno Schenk adds Clement, the scholia on Germanicus,[85] and a number of the Roman poets: he discounts the role Reifferscheid also assigned certain lost works of

---

[84] Brehaut, *op. cit.*, p. 47.

[85] Arno Schenk, *De Isidori Hispalensis de natura rerum libelli fontibus* (Jena, 1909). Stahl, *op. cit.*, p. 123, states that Isidore made use of Suetonius' lost encyclopedia which he thought a translation of a late Greek effort, but adduces no evidence for this view.

Suetonius.[86] Laistner adds Gregory the Great, Placidus, Donatus, Victorinus, the logical and scientific writings of Boethius, Gargilius Martialis, Palladius and the agrimensores.[87] Varro is often cited by name as an authority.[88] Laistner notes:

As to the numerous citations from poets and from Republican prose writers, while Isidore was familiar with some at first hand, like Virgil and Lucan, and perhaps Ovid, Juvenal, Martial, and Sallust, the rest, especially citations from early authors like Ennius, Plautus, the Roman writers of tragedy, Lucilius, and Cato, were copied by him from his sources.[89]

Lindsay's list of citations is seven pages long, and includes seventy-three authors, ranging from Caesar Grammaticus to Petronius Arbiter, but again, the extent of Isidore's familiarity with their writings at first hand must remain uncertain.[90]

Within the narrow limits of general encyclopedia articles on medicine for laymen, Isidore is a conscientious and reliable informant who borrowed the medical portions of his *Etymologiae* intelligently enough to present a brief but tolerably complete survey of the medical learning of his time. Fletcher observes:

The library of Isidore was contained in fourteen *armaria* (presses) adorned with the portraits of twenty-two authors. From the elegaic verses which Isidore wrote to commemorate these authors, we learn that over the press containing the medical MSS. were the portraits of SS. Cosmas and Damian, Hippocrates and Galen. The SS. were patrons of the art of medicine, not authors, as far as we know, but the choice of Hippocrates and Galen show a critical discernment. Isidore unfortunately gives us no list of his medical books, but shall we be far wrong in thinking that, following Cassiodorus in many things, he had among others collected the works recommended by that Father to his monks. Dioscorides, Hippocrates, Galen *Ad Glauconem,* all of which were to be had in Latin translations, Caelius Aurelianus or possibly Celsus. Who was the anonymous author possessed by Cassiodorus? Possibly the Compendium of Oribasius or that of Cassius Felix. Isidore certainly possessed a copy of Cassius, but I am doubtful about Oribasius, and think that Isidore's source of Galen was an

epitome of that author corresponding to those found in the middle ages.[91]

In both Caelius Aurelianus and Cassius Felix, discussion of specific diseases proceeds in the traditional head-to-foot sequence. Isidore seems to lean heavily on material much like that of Caelius Aurelianus, although not so heavily as Drabkin suggests,[92] and it is not clear whether Isidore knew Caelius Aurelianus in full—perhaps in fuller form than has survived—or in abridgment, or both. *Etymologiae* IV reflects two distinct schools of medical thinking, but this is more apt to stem from the medical writings available than from meditated choice. The Methodist sect, represented by Caelius Aurelianus, seems to have been the source for most of his descriptions of acute and chronic diseases in chapters six and seven, and the Logical or Dogmatic sect, represented more typically by Hippocrates, Galen and Cassius Felix, provides the bulk of the remaining properly medical material. Pharmacology and materia medica resemble the tradition of Pliny and Dioscorides, and may include material derived from Theophrastus. This defines Isidore's sources less than suggests their kind. There are echoes in a discussion of the plague of writers as diverse as Pseudo-Clement and Lucretius; of scabies and leprosy from Leviticus; of musical therapy from Cassiodorus and of cancer from Augustine of Hippo. *Etymologiae* XI, which discusses man and his parts, contains much material similar to that in Lactantius, Ambrose, Tertullian, and the Servian Vergil Commentaries, but whether Isidore used the Servian Commentaries or whether he used common material remains conjectural.[93] Whether or not Quintus Serenus Sammonicus, Scribonius Largus, and Theodore Priscan can be considered sources remains equally conjectural for the same reason. A very large number of medical and anatomical terms and definitions have been drawn from nonmedical literature: Cicero, Seneca, Plato, Varro, Verrius Flac-

---

[86] A. Reifferscheid, *C. Suetoni Tranquilli praeter Caesarum libros reliquiae* (Leipzig, 1860) considers the *Etymologiae* neither more nor less than an Isidorian reworking of a lost Latin encyclopedia.

[87] Laistner, *op. cit.,* p. 93.

[88] H. Kettner, *Varronische studien* (Halle, 1865) discusses Varro's influence on the *Etymologiae,* and see IV. 8. 13; IV. 11. 15; XI. 1. 51; XI. 1. 97 and XI. 3. 1.

[89] Laistner, *op. cit.,* pp. 93–94.

[90] W. M. Lindsay, *Isidori Hispalensis episcopi Etymologiarum sive Originum libri* (2 v., Oxford, 1911). The text is unpaginated: the *loci citati* are at the end of the second volume, but this list includes only authors cited by name. Stahl, *op.cit.,* pp. 215–216, points out that Isidore does not cite, by name, such writers as Tertullian, Cassiodorus, Solinus, or Servius. Whether or not Isidore used the Servian Commentaries is not clear, he certainly used similar material, but he probably was indebted to Tertullian, Cassiodorus, and Solinus, so that this list is strictly of citations and not of putative sources. See note 93, below.

[91] Fletcher, *op. cit.,* p. 86. The verses, almost surely apocryphal, said to have been inscribed by Isidore above the cases in his library are printed, in slightly different versions, by C. H. Beeson, *op. cit.,* pp. 157–166, and by Karl Sudhoff, "Die verse Isidors von Sevilla auf dem Schrank der medizinischen Werke seiner Bibliothek," *Mitteilungen zur Geschichte der Medizin und der Naturwissenschaften* 15 (1915) : 200.

[92] I. E. Drabkin, *Caelius Aurelianus on Acute Diseases and on Chronic Diseases* (Chicago, 1950), p. xv.

[93] Fletcher, *op. cit.,* p. 78, points out thirty-three apparent references from Servius in *Etymologiae* IV and XI, although Nettleship (*Lectures and essays* [Oxford, 1885], pp. 329–330) believes that Servius and Isidore use a common source, perhaps Verrius Flaccus: "I think, and will endeavour to show, that Isidore did not copy from the vulgate of Servius, but that the numerous coincidences between the vulgate and Isidore are due to community of sources, and also that a comparison between Isidore and the fuller Servius shows that many notes in the latter are absolutely homogeneous with the vulgate, and cannot, therefore, be supposed to be interpolations." This writer agrees with Nettleship, but for differing views, see Stahl, *loc. cit.,* and George Homeyer, *De scholiis Vergilianis Isidori fontibus* (Jena, 1913), pp. 84–85.

cus, Vergil, and the Servian Commentaries, Ovid, Horace and many others have been suggested but again, proof is difficult.[94]

ISIDORE'S PHYSICAL UNIVERSE

A common view of the physical universe was accepted in late classical and patristic times in its broad outline as the simplest explanation for data whose evaluation was limited by, among other things, the parameters of the unaided human senses and by a mathematics which did not effectively progress beyond arithmetic and geometry. This view of the world underlay ancient scientific thinking, and reflected itself in medical and anatomic terms no less than in philosophical and cosmological schemata. Francis Adams of Banchory sums this up:

Contrary, then, to what is very generally supposed, it would appear that there was at bottom no very great difference of opinion between the philosophers of the Ionic school and those of other sects, namely, the Pythagoreans, Platonists, Peripatetics, Stoics, and Epicureans; and further, that, from the earliest dawn of philosophy, down to the time when it fell into neglect and came to be misunderstood, the physical doctrines of the philosophers underwent but little variation.[95]

In this view of the universe, all elements are modifications of a primary common substance itself devoid of quality and form but susceptible of assuming all forms and qualities—whether the primary substance be the eternal chaos of the Stoics, the shapeless mass of Aristotle or the self-existing atoms of Democritus.

Empedocles of Agrigentum, during the fifth century B.C., had explained the constitution of matter in terms of four qualities—heat, cold, dryness, and moisture—active in the human body as in all created things. Greek medical theories arising after the time of the Hippocratic school came to be based on these four elemental qualities, with their corresponding bodily humors. Pythagoras may earlier have taught that the health of a human body depends upon a proper balance between its component parts, and the Pythagorean Philolaus, in the fifth century B.C., is said to have explained disease as a disturbance among the elements which form the bodily humors. These men, like the Ionian philosophers generally, were not physicians and their deductions were based on theoretical considerations rather than clinical observation. Transformations among the elements themselves arise from combinations among the basic qualities: hotness, dryness, coldness, and wetness. An example is change in the physical state of water with changes in temperature:

Hot and Dry	Hot and Wet	Cold and Wet	Cold and Dry
AIR ⇌	STEAM ⇌	WATER ⇌	ICE

Plato called the four elements postulated by the Pythagoreans *stoicheia*, a word latinized to *elementa*. The four primary elements are arranged in layers according to their weights, each with typical qualities shading gradually into the others to produce the vast variety of creation, each stratum with its own inhabitants. Later thinkers specified these inhabitants: in the fiery heavens, from which the celestial bodies drew their light, lived the angels;[96] in the air, birds and spirits; in the water, fishes; while the solid earth of which the world is mainly composed was the habitation of animals and men.[97] According to Isidore, these elements are in constant flux between the earth and the solar fire, much as Lucretius and the Greek cosmologists had taught:

Concerning the Elements: HYLÊ is the Greek word for a certain primary material of things, directly formed in no shape, but capable of all bodily forms, from which these visible elements are shaped, and it is from this derivation that they get their names. This *HYLÊ* the Latins have called "matter," *materia*, because although altogether formless, that from which anything is made is always termed "matter." For this reason also poets have named it "timber," *silva*, not inappropriately, because materials, *materiae*, are of timber. The Greeks, however, have named the elements *STOICHEIA* because they come together by a certain commingling and concordance of association. They are thus said to be joined among themselves by a certain natural proportion, [so that] something originating in the form of fire returns again to earth, and from earth to fire just as, for example, fire ends in air, air is condensed into water, water thickens into earth; and earth is again dissolved into water, water evaporates into air, air is reduced into fire. Therefore it is that all elements are present in all things, but the name is derived from the one which it has in greater quantity. Moreover, they are divided by divine providence among proper inhabitants: the Creator Himself has filled heaven with angels, the air with birds, the sea with fishes and the earth with men and other animals.[98]

In his discussion of the parts of the human body, Isidore states:

But flesh is composed of four elements: earth is in the fleshy parts, air in the breath, water in the blood, fire in the vital heat. The elements are mingled in us in their proper proportions, of which something is lacking when the conjunction is dissolved.[99]

The four humors are related to the four elements, and each humor has a corresponding element which shares its qualities: blood, like air, is hot and moist; yellow bile is hot and dry, like fire; black bile is cold and dry like earth; and phlegm is cold and wet like water. This humoral pathology originated before the time of the Hippocratic school, and under the influence of

---

[94] Enrico Dressel, "De Isidori Originum fontibus," *Rivista di Filologia e d'Istruzione Classica* 3 (1874–1875): 263.

[95] Francis Adams, *The Genuine Works of Hippocrates* (London, 1849) 2: p. 147.

[96] For Aristotle's views on the ether, see *De generatione et corruptione* 2. 8 [334b30–335a5]. Ambrose uses *STOICHEIA* as *elementa*, e.g., *Hexameron* 3. 4. 18 [PL 14: 164].

[97] Cicero, *De natura deorum* 2. 33.

[98] XIII. 3. 1–3; see also his *De natura rerum* 11. 1. Souter lists *silva* as a synonym for *materia*, *HYLÊ*, in Chalcidius' *Commentarius in Platonis Timaeum*.

[99] XI. 1. 16.

SOUTH

```
        DRYNESS                                HEAT

              FIRE
             SUMMER
           YELLOW BILE
            CHOLERIC

    EARTH       Element       AIR
   AUTUMN       Season      SPRING
W  BLACK BILE   Humor        BLOOD    E
E  MELANCHOLIC  Temperament  SANGUINE A
S                                     S
T                                     T

              WATER
             WINTER
             PHLEGM
            PHLEGMATIC
        COLDNESS                           MOISTURE
```

NORTH

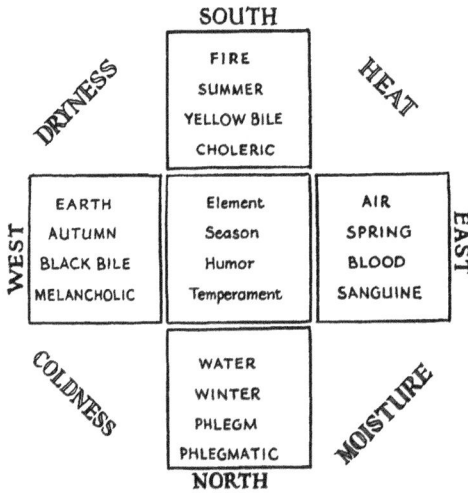

SCHEMA OF THE FOUR ELEMENTS

and their distribution in the world, year, human body and its temperaments, quarters of the globe and prevailing winds according to Isidore of Seville.

Galen and his followers, remained a dominant force in normal and pathologic physiology for centuries.

These humors were formed and renewed daily under the influence of many factors, all of which were to be carefully considered in assessment of their disorders: the season of the year, the patient's age, prevailing winds, local rainfall and temperature fluctuations, the degree of sunlight and shadow, the patient's diet and habits. Different humors dominated successive stages of life: blood in youth, yellow bile in early manhood, black bile in middle age, and phlegm in old age. The bodily constitution is determined by the proportions in which these elemental qualities are mixed, the *temperamentum*. Health consists in a harmony of these elements, and excess or defect in one or more of these qualities produces disease. Acute diseases develop from hot humors, and chronic diseases from the cold: humoral disharmonies in any part affect the whole body through disruption of the delicate humoral balance, and rational therapy restores this balance by the removal or neutralization of the peccant humor, whether by bleeding, purging, sweating, or vomiting, or through the use of internal or external medications.

Isidore explains meteorological no less than medical phenomena in terms of the four elements: the upper air, like the fire above it, is calm and cloudless; the lower air is cloudy and disturbed from association with

the element water.[100] Clouds are composed of condensed water which may further condense to form rain.[101] With regard to the seasons of the year, spring is hot and moist; summer hot and dry; autumn dry and cold; winter cold and moist.[102] The points of the compass are related to the seasons and to the elements, the winds to the elements and through them, to the four humors of the body and their varying domination not only at different ages of life but at different seasons of the year. This explains, in part, ancient medical concern with the influence of winds, geographic location and seasons on the human body.[103]

The Galenic humoral pathology has been summarized by Professor Major Greenwood:

. . . a less intelligent physician than Galen would have perceived that human temperaments, psychological and corporal, vary and that temperament is a factor of medical prophylaxis, diagnosis and treatment. The traditional doctrine of opposite qualities—the hot and the cold, the moist and the dry—he used as a frame of reference. For him, every human temperament could be represented by a point in a plane the position of which is determined by its coordinates (the origin is the ideal point, the perfect crasis). So the universe of human temperaments will be a frequency surface in the statistical sense. Galen did not, of course, express this geometrically but verbally and verbosely. His successors ignored his insistence on continuity and picked out "typical" temperaments; hence one has the nine temperaments, viz. the perfect temperament, denoted in Galen's system by a point, the four simple excesses, denoted by points on the axes, viz.

$$(+x, 0)\ (-x, 0)\ (0, +y)\ (0, -y)$$

and the four linked excesses, viz. all the points in the four quadrants. Even this was too much, the nine temperaments dwindled into four, the choleric, sanguine, phlegmatic and melancholic, which survived the oblivion of the humours and qualities and still live. Galen's insistence on continuity was forgotten by clinicians.[104]

Although very superficially, this humoral system did explain clinical data. There was no ancient pathology: the ancient and medieval physician studied nosology, the symptoms of disease, and prognosis, its natural history and probable course in any particular patient. Symptoms were treated as though they were the disease, and an accurate analysis of this ancient nosologic reasoning is given by a modern pathologist:

The Greeks related their theory of disease to the fact that the blood separated into layers when obtained from sick patients, the four humours being represented by these separated parts of the blood. The sedimented red cells can be divided into a dark or "melancholic" humour and a red or "sanguine" humour, depending on the degree of oxygenation, while the upper cell-free fibrin clot constituted the phlegmatic and the supernatant serum the choleric humour. It was not unnatural to suppose that this separa-

---

[100] XIII. 7. 1.
[101] XIII. 7. 2.
[102] V. 35. 1; Isidore, *De natura rerum* 7. 4.
[103] IV. 13. 3.
[104] Major Greenwood, *Authority in Medicine: Old and New* (Cambridge, 1943), pp. 24–25.

tion, apparently due to an abnormal increase of one of the humours, was the cause rather than the result of illness, and hence that the removal of the abnormal humour by bleeding would be likely to restore health.[105]

Empedocles' theory of the four elemental qualities was influential enough, but his adoption of the primitive notion that the blood is the seat of the *thermon emphyton*, the "inner heat" necessary for life was equally important.[106] This made the heart the center of the vascular tree, the chief organ for the distribution of the *pneuma*, variably identified as "air" or "breath." Observing that every organ has a branching system of veins, arteries, and nerves plaited together, Erasistratos of Chios, in the third century B.C., concluded that their minutest branches formed the tissues. Blood, carried through the veins, and the two kinds of *pneuma*, provided for nutrition and motion: air was taken in by the lungs and passed to the heart, there becoming the vital spirit, the *pneuma zôtikon*, to be sent in turn to the body through the arteries; carried to the brain, it became the animal spirit, the *pneuma psychikon*, and was distributed to various parts of the body through the nerves, which were thought to be hollow, possibly because of the nutrient arteries which accompany the major nerve trunks and which are empty after death, to produce thought and organic movement. Galen later taught that the chyle was brought from the digestive tract by the portal vessels to the liver and was there endowed with *pneuma* to become the natural spirit, the *pneuma physikon*, which was distributed by the veins, ebbing and flooding from the liver which was the seat of the body's heat. Practically speaking, the *pneuma* seemed to pass through the arteries which are empty at death, although Galen taught that they contained blood during life. The pneumatic theory was also, in part, a Stoic attempt to reconcile divergent philosophical approaches to physiology: the individual's *pneuma* reflected the world *pneuma* and, seated in the thorax, was the vital spark for all physiological functions.[107]

Isidore flatly denies that the human soul is part of the world *pneuma*:

The soul is not a part of the divine substance, or Nature; it does not exist before the body is formed, but it is created at the same time as the body, to which it seems to be bound. The opinions of the philosophers hold that the soul exists before it is born in the body. But there is no proof of this, for whether or not we existed before, we neither know ourselves nor do we have any man who can tell us. Let us therefore not seek for what is so ridiculous.[108]

Galen taught that both ventricles of the heart, arteries, and veins contained blood, but lacking knowledge of the capillaries, he was unable to formulate a coherent theory of the circulation. He himself does not seem to have identified the *pneuma* with air, or to have thought that it circulated in the arteries, but he did teach that the pulse distributed the innate heat from the heart to the other parts of the body, and nourished the *pneuma zôtikon*, or vital spirit. Both Galen and Aristotle interpreted the superior and inferior venae cavae as arising from the liver and only incidentally opening into the right atrium during their course. A recent writer comments:

Galen . . . held that the source of the *pneuma psychikon* was internal and that it arose as an exhalation of the blood. The blood exhaled this *pneuma* under the influence of the innate heat. He says: "But if the breath of the blood is required for the nutrition of the *pneuma psychikon* (for it is reasonable that this is so), healthy animals would receive the greatest value from moderate heat. For how would cold blood be released into breath? But moderately warm blood can easily be scattered in cloudy and smoky vapours." (Galen, *De utilitate respirationis* 5 [Kühn 4:506–507].)
A paramount influence is thus given to the *innate heat*, and Galen makes clear that he regards the principal function of the respiration to be the maintenance of the innate heat.[109]

As noted, Isidore locates the element air in the breath, but elemental fire in the vital heat.[110]

ISIDORE AND THE MICROCOSM

Isidore holds the traditional philosophical notion that each individual human being is a microcosm within himself, paralleling the universe, the macrocosm, on a miniature scale. He is composed of the same four elements, distributed in much the same manner as in the universe: all things exist in him, and just as the universe is explicable in terms of man, man is explicable in terms of the universe. The finer details of this theory of micro-macrocosmic parallelism varied from time to time and from thinker to thinker, but its broad outlines dominated patristic and medieval cosmology. According to this hypothesis, man alone integrates within himself all the constituents of reality and man is the connecting link between the material and spiritual worlds. Man forms the central link in the great chain of being: this anthropocentricity does not infer that the universe exists for the sake of man but that man is the key to the whole cosmic riddle, and that insight into human nature will provide insight into that of the universe. Plato seems to interpret the macrocosm as an enlargement of an anthropocentric microcosm, and to have assumed the existence of a world soul as the principle of order and growth within the universe. According to Plato's theory, man

[105] R. G. Macfarlane, "Reactions of the Blood to Injury," in Howard Florey, ed., *Lectures on General Pathology* (London, 1954), p. 219.
[106] Pseudo-Soranus, *Quaestiones medicinales* 66 [Rose 256].
[107] Some medieval thinkers identified the "world soul" of the Neoplatonic philosophers, the *anima mundi*, with the third person of the Trinity, the *spiritus sanctus*, a view condemned in 1121 by the Council of Soissons.
[108] Isidore, *Sententiarum* I. 12. 4 [*PL* 83: 562–563].

[109] L. G. Wilson, "Erasistratus, Galen and the *Pneuma*," *Bulletin of the History of Medicine* 33 (1959): 293, discusses Galen's theory of the *pneuma*; the quotation is at p. 311.
[110] XI. 1. 16.

creates other orderly worlds (political, artistic, and the like) around himself, each of which—in a certain manner—reflects this basic world order.

The terms *microcosm* and *macrocosm* appear later than their corresponding ideas: in the New Academy and among the Stoics, man was often spoken of as the *brachus kosmos*, the "little universe."[111] The Greek fathers use the terms almost without explanation, and apparently consider them well-enough known to make comment superfluous. Although their sources were doubtless Neoplatonic, Latin writers depend chiefly on such later authorities as Macrobius and Chalcidius' *Commentary on the Timaeus*. Isidore's authority contributed to the wide acceptance of the concept in the West.[112] Plato presents most of his views on the world-soul in the *Timaeus*,[113] but neither there nor in the *Philebus* does he maintain that the individual soul is part of, or originates with, the world-soul. This is a later development, and a still later extension of microcosmism held that man includes within himself the whole universe through his knowledge of it, and that although complete knowledge may indeed exist only as a theoretical possibility, remote and unattainable, the human mind and, through it man, becomes the whole universe and thereby, all things.[114]

Although this microcosmism underwent certain variations, it maintained a remarkable continuity. Rudolf Allers epitomizes this:

The idea that the universe is animated becomes with many, especially medieval, writers the reason for calling man the microscosm and for comparing the universe to man. Thus it had been with Philo, thus it remained through many centuries. Man is the true image of the universe because both are animated by souls. The rationality of the World-Soul had been stressed by Macrobius and became a generally accepted doctrine. The World-Soul is gifted with rationality, and the human souls, derived from the former, owe to it their rational powers. They stand to their bodies much in the same relation as the World-Soul to the universe, insofar as both are governing principles of their respective "bodies." Then, the micro-macrocosmic parallel becomes inescapable. Numenius ascribes such a view to Plato. This view, however, endangers the uniqueness of the human person and was, accordingly, deemed inacceptable by several of the earlier Scholastics.[115]

Medieval philosophical thought provided a foundation for every intellectual and mystical endeavor, speculative or not, linking all knowledge from the greatest

to the least in dignity: ethics and medicine, metaphysics and anatomy each had a settled position in this hierarchy of knowledge. Isidore thus describes man:

He has in himself something of fire, of air, of water and of earth. The proportion of earth is in the flesh; of water in the blood; of air in the breath; of fire in the vital heat. For thus the fourfold ratio of the human body marks out the appearance of the four elements. The head refers to the heavens, in which are located the two eyes, like the lights of the sun and moon. The breath is joined to the air, because just as the breath of respiration is sent thence, so also the blasts of wind come from the air. The belly is compared to the sea, because of a collection of all of the humors, like a gathering together of waters. Finally, the soles of the feet are compared to [the element] earth, since the extremities of the members are dry, or parched, as is also the earth. For truly, the mind is located in the eminence of the head, as God is in heaven, so that He may survey and govern all things from on high.[116]

Much later in the Middle Ages, Robert Grosseteste of Lincoln (*ca.* 1175–1253) applied this doctrine to the human body in almost identical terms.[117]

In providing etymologies for the names of the parts of the human body, Isidore was guided not only by the doctrine of the microcosm, but by a grammatical tradition which required an interpretation of even anatomic terms over and above their logical meanings. In Isidore's time, the grammarian's dignity approached that of the metaphysician, and naming an object was often the first step toward understanding it, a powerful impetus to the compilation of an encyclopedia based on etymologies. Isidore often provides etymologies unrelated to the real functions of the body's parts, yet just such etymologies were commonplace in the standard medical works of such writers as Pseudo-Soranus and Cassius. Isidore conscientiously attempts to define and distinguish medical terms analogically with regard to their utility to the individual, and for Isidore, utility can be esthetic or symbolic as well as functional.[118]

ISIDORE AND THE *HĒGEMONIKON*

Isidore's psychology is concerned with the functions of the soul, and reflects the views of the patristic period, with its traditional cerebral localization of function. Important in this is the concept of the *hēgemonikon* which Isidore assumes rather than develops. Tertullian had stated,

At the beginning, we must decide whether there is in the soul some supreme principle of life and intelligence,

---

[111] Aristotle, *Physica* 8. 2 [252b26].

[112] On the role of the *Timaeus* and its commentators in forming Isidore's intellectual milieu, see Fontaine, *op. cit.*, pp. 579–580, who discusses Isidore's interpretation of the microcosm at pp. 662 ff.

[113] Plato, *Timaeus* 34B; and see A. E. Taylor, *Plato: the Man and His Work* (London, 1949), pp. 440 ff.

[114] Aristotle, *De anima* 3. 8 [431b21]: this is what this writer means when he says that the human soul is πῶς ἀπάντα "as it were, everything." See Thomas Aquinas, *In III de Anima* 1. 13 and *Summa Theologica* 1 q. 84, a. 2 ad sec.

[115] Rudolf Allers, *op. cit.*, pp. 345–346, traces the development of the microcosmic theory.

[116] Isidore, *Differentiarum* II. 48–49 [*PL* 83: 77–78].

[117] Robert Grosseteste, "Quod homo sit minor mundus," in L. Baur, "Die Philosophie des Robert Grosseteste," *Beiträge zur Geschichte der Philosophie des Mittelalters* 9 (1912): 59. There is an English translation in C. G. Wallis, *Giovanni Pico Della Mirandola, The Very Elegant Speech on the Dignity of Man* (Annapolis, 1949), p. 25.

[118] Fontaine, *op. cit.*, pp. 666–668, discusses this problem in detail.

the so-called *hêgemonikon* or directing principle. Otherwise, the very existence of the soul is called in question.[119]

Pseudo-Soranus had defined the *hêgemonikon* as "the chief principle of the soul, presiding over the whole body and, residing in the brain, ruling over the whole body."[120] Tertullian dissented, and placed the soul in the region of the heart:

Hence, one cannot agree with Heraclitus that the principal part of the soul can be stirred from without, nor with Moschion that it is somehow diffused throughout the whole body. Plato [*Timaeus* 69D] also is wrong when he says the soul is in the head, as well as Xenocrates, who thought it was in the crown of the head. It does not repose in the brain, as Hippocrates taught, nor around the base of the brain, according to Herophilus. Strato and Erasistratus erred in saying that it was in the outer membranes of the brain. Strato, the physician, wrongly placed it between the eyebrows. Epicurus says the soul lies within the structure of the breast. The truth is rather to be found among the Egyptians, especially in the writings of those among them who knew Holy Scripture. There is a verse of Orpheus or Empedocles which reads: "The seat of sensation lies in the blood around the heart."[121]

Lactantius was uncertain as to the soul's location, debating between the brain and "that two-fold division of blood which is enclosed by the heart,"[122] and concluding:

But at the summit of that fabrication of His, which we have said to be very like the keel of a ship [the spine], He has placed the head, in which is located the rule [*regimen*] of every living thing; and this name has been given it, as Varro once wrote to Cicero, because sensation and nerves have their beginnings there.[123]

Lactantius located the soul thus on entirely *a priori* grounds: the highest part of the body is the most dignified and all sensation centers there,[124] but he denies that there is a pathway from the brain to the thorax.[125]

Tertullian had noted, "the soul is so united to the mind that they are not distinct substances, but . . . the mind is a faculty of the soul."[126] The notion of "mind," *mens*, in early Christian Latin writers is precisely equivalent to the Greek *nous*, as that word was

used by late Hellenistic philosophical writers. Tertullian explains this:

By "mind," I mean merely that faculty which is inherent and implanted in the soul and proper to it by birth and by which the soul acts and gains knowledge. The possession of this faculty makes it possible for the soul to act upon itself, the soul being moved by the mind as if they were different substances.[127]

This traditional psychology defined the difference between sensation and thought, and distinguished between error and illusion. Again citing Tertullian:

The Epicureans with complete consistency maintain that the senses always report the truth, but they explain the illusions in a way different from the Stoics. In their opinion, the senses report the truth, but our minds lead us astray. The function of the senses is to receive an impression, not to think; that is the function of the soul. They deny to the senses the power of thinking and to the soul all power of sensation.[128]

Tertullian identified the vital spirit with the soul, a position which Isidore and most orthodox Christians rejected because they thought it close to pantheism— of which, indeed, Tertullian has been accused.[129] Most early Christian writers were sufficiently impressed by contemporary theories to reject the Old Testament localization of the soul in the blood.[130] Isidore does not assign any bodily part as the soul's habitat, but looks upon the soul as the incorporeal part of man, his *hêgemonikon*.

ISIDORE'S ANATOMY AND PHYSIOLOGY

Isidore's treatment of anatomy and physiology is less technical than his discussion of properly medical topics, and reflects little more than the notions current among literate laymen of his time. Strongly teleological, *Etymologiae* XI sometimes amounts to nothing more than a list of anatomical examples to document

---

[119] Tertullian, *De anima* 15. 1 [Waszink 18], translation by Quain, *op. cit.*, p. 209.

[120] Pseudo-Soranus, *Quaestiones medicinales* 70 [Rose 256].

[121] Tertullian, *De anima* 15. 5 [Waszink 19]; translation by Quain, *op. cit.*, pp. 210–211. See also H. B. Brown, "The Anatomical Habitat of the Soul," *Annals of Medical History* 5 (1923): 1.

[122] Lactantius, *De opificio Dei* 16 [*CSEL* 27: 53]: *aut in medulla cerebri haereat aut in illo sanguine bipartito qui est conclusus in corde.* This apparently refers to the two sides of the heart, since the ancients considered the atrium and ventricle together a single chamber.

[123] Lactantius, *De opificio Dei* 5 [*CSEL* 27: 20].

[124] Lactantius, *De opificio Dei* 16 [*CSEL* 27: 52].

[125] Lactantius, *De opificio Dei* 16 [*CSEL* 27: 53]: *ad pectus ex cerebro nullum iter pateat.*

[126] Tertullian, *De anima* 12. 6 [Waszink 17]; translation by Quain, *op. cit.*, p. 206.

[127] Tertullian, *De anima* 12. 1 [Waszink 16]; translation by Quain, *op. cit.*, p. 205.

[128] Tertullian, *De anima* 17. 4 [Waszink 22]; translation by Quain, *op. cit.*, p. 215.

[129] Tertullian, *De anima* 10. 2 [Waszink 12] equates the breath and the soul. This is rejected by Isidore, who considers the soul an incorporeal substance and not a breath of air. Quain, *op. cit.*, p. 199, notes: "Because of his belief that the soul was the 'breath of God' (relying on Gen. 2. 7) and the concomitance of life and breathing, Tertullian assumed that the soul was breath, i.e., some tenuous form of airy substance."

Isidore considered Tertullian in error when he asserted, *De anima* 10. 9 [Waszink 14]: *ipse erit anima spiritus, sicut, ipsa dies lux. Ipsum est enim quid, per quod est quid.* "The soul is the breath just as day is the light [of day] itself. There is no difference between a being and that by which it is a being." At *De anima* 11. 1 [Waszink 14]: "The soul is a spirit because it respires and not because it is actually a 'spirit.' Breathing and respiration are the same thing. Since one of the properties of the soul is respiration, we are forced to call the soul a spirit." (Translation by Quain, *op. cit.*, p. 202). See Isidore, XI. 1. 10.

[130] See Genesis 9: 1–7 and Leviticus 17: 11.

the beneficence of God. Despite the theological bias of Ambrose and Lactantius and the literary flavor of the Servian Vergil commentaries, there are passages of genuine value to the historian of science. In his anatomical portions, although accurate as far as they go, Isidore is less concerned with logical definitions than with correlation between structure and function in the light of etymologies to explain the body's utility, whether esthetic, functional, or symbolic. The difference between *Etymologiae* XI, "On Man and Monsters," and *Etymologiae* IV, "On Medicine," is, in part, the difference between a general and a medical dictionary.

He notes that many useful parts of the body are beautiful, such as the hands and feet, but that other parts, like the viscera, are merely useful.[131] He does not develop an evolutionary theory in any modern sense of the word but he believes that useful differences may evolve to produce harmony between structure and function and thereby to manifest the wisdom of God no less than through direct creation: it is to facilitate carrying and bearing young, for example, that women's hips are wider than men's.[132] His discussion of man and his parts begins with the observation that nature is the power of making and of begetting, which some identify with God.[133] Man was created from the earth,[134] and stands erect even though his body is made from earth since he is composed of body and soul.[135]

For Isidore, man is two-fold, composed of body and soul. The soul, although incorporeal, is not air since it exists while the human being is still in his mother's womb and cannot breathe. He notes that the "soul" is sometimes spoken of as though it were the "breath" or vital spirit, as in various passages in Scripture. The mind is a function of the soul, but pertains to thought and not to life as such, since even the mindless are alive. The intellect knows and reasons.[136] Isidore thus summarizes the traditional teaching on the faculties of the soul:

The memory is also the intellect, and for this reason those who are forgetful are "mindless." When it gives life to the body, it is the soul; when it wills, it is the mind; when it knows, it is the intellect; when it remembers, it is the memory; when it judges correctly, it is the reason; when it breathes, it is the vital spirit; when it perceives anything, it is sensation.[137]

The names of the faculties of the soul are assigned only for convenience in discussion, and the soul remains a unity.[138]

Unlike some early Christian writers who denigrated the human body to the extent of denying that the human

being was more than a soul, Isidore insists that man is both body and soul, although it is the soul which was created in the image of God:

Man's soul is not the man, but the body—which was made from dust—is just as much man. By living in the body, however, by that very participation in human flesh, the soul is named, just as the Apostle said that the inner man, the soul, not the flesh, was made in the image of God. It is wrongly believed by some that the human soul is corporeal because it was made in the image of God, as though God were not immutable; neverthless, it is as incorporeal as God.[139]

For Isidore, although the words may look alike, "mind" (*animus*) and "soul" (*anima*) differ in their meanings:

There is this difference between "mind," *animus*, and "soul," *anima:* the mind pertains to the judgment and the soul to life; the latter is always the same, the former is changed according to mood. Likewise, the ancients distinguished "intellect," *mens*, from mind: intellect, as they understood it, was really the mind as it willed, or as it was able to learn. Moreover, sometimes "mind" is said for "energy," *vis.*[140]

Isidore neither underestimates the importance of man's will nor overlooks conflict between opposing desires of flesh and spirit;

Learned men have said that there is this difference between the soul, *anima*, and the vital spirit, *spiritus*, because the soul itself is man's life, presiding over the body's sensation and motion; the vital spirit of the soul itself is whatever energy and rational potency it has, through which, by the law of nature, it seems to excel over other animals. For this reason, the soul is the breath of life, making man an animal, but the vital spirit is the force which suppresses carnal desires, and stirs up mortal man for the goal of an immortal life.[141]

Carnal and spiritual desires are only a part, a function, of the vital spirit, whether understood as libido or concupiscence:

There is this difference between concupiscence of the flesh and the vital spirit: concupiscence of the flesh is a motion of a sinful soul as a result of squalid dilectation; but concupiscence of the vital spirit is an ardent intention of the mind upon desires for holy virtue. Those consenting to the latter send themselves to the Kingdom, to the former, to eternal torture. The former is the law of sin, descending from the damnation of the first man, the latter is the law of intelligence, proceeding from the gift of our Redeemer.[142]

Turning from the soul to the body, Isidore proceeds in a systematic head-to-foot sequence, with an occasional digression. The head is the most important part of the body, and is provided with hair both for ornament and for protection.[143] The face not only enables us to recognize one another, but expresses age, personality, and state of mind, and in a very special way, the eyes

---

131 XI. 1. 146.
132 XI. 1. 147.
133 XI. 1. 1.
134 XI. 1. 2–4.
135 XI. 1. 4, 5–7, 109.
136 XI. 1. 6–12.
137 XI. 1. 13.
138 XI. 1. 12.

---

139 Isidore, *Sententiarum* I. 12. 2 [*PL* 83: 562].
140 Isidore, *Differentiarum* I. 37 [*PL* 83: 14].
141 Isidore, *Differentiarum* II. 98 [*PL* 83: 84].
142 Isidore, *Differentiarum* II, 109 [*PL* 83: 86].
143 XI. 1. 28.

reveal much about the soul and inner character.[144] The eyes are carefully protected by their position deep within the skull, and loss of their normal luster can be a sign of approaching death.[145] Much attention is given to the etymologies of the major bones of the skull, and to their functions.

Hearing is the work of the ear, and Isidore's account may conceal a reference to the bony labyrinth, but it is so vague that certainty is impossible on this point.[146] Olfaction proceeds from odors carried by the air, and the nose and its parts are described.[147] Speech is produced by the motion of the tongue against the teeth, "like the plectrum of a stringed instrument," and it is observed that if the tongue is immobile, only a single tone can be produced. The teeth are described and classified as incisors, canines, and molars, and the gums both grow teeth and form an ornament to soften the appearance of these bare bones.[148] Vision is the most powerful of the senses and sight results from a union between lucid spirits proceeding both from the eye and from the object perceived: this perception is a function of the brain, and does not take place in the eye itself.[149] The sensation described as touch can arise inside or from without the body.[150] All sensation is relayed through the nerves to the head, whence the body is governed and where all the nerves have their beginnings.[151]

The bones are the foundation of the body: the word used in their description suggests that they serve as the foundation of a building.[152] The function of tendons and their role in motion and in the skeletal articulations are appreciated.[153] Cartilage is admirably described with reference to its function in articular surfaces and in places requiring strength combined with flexibility.[154] The bone marrow is thought to moisten and nourish the bones.[155] The structure of the bony spine and sacrum is discussed,[156] and the function of the spinal cord as a part of the central nervous system is clearly defined and described as an extension of the brain which passes through the spinal canal.[157] The anatomy of the hip joint is accurately described,[158] and the structure of the foot is discussed at considerable length.[159]

Isidore's account of the skeleton is less osteologic than topographic, and is more concerned with surface relationships than with details of skeletal structure. The neck, for example, is compared to a column which supports the head much as a pillar supports its capitol.[160] The limbs are provided with various etymologies in the light of their functions. The hand is discussed in great symbolic and functional detail, and each of the fingers is assigned a proper name and etymology—respectively, thumb, index finger, lewd finger, ring finger or medicinal finger, and auricular finger, the latter because "we scratch our ears with it." [161] The limits of the trunk are defined, and the thorax is compared to an ark or stronghold for the protection of the vital organs within.[162] The ribs, sides, and back are discussed with fanciful etymologies and many references to comparable organs in lower animals.[163] The buttocks, as an example, are fleshy so that the bones do not feel pain from the weight of the body when seated.[164]

Viscera is a general term applied to all of the body's parts, and is not restricted to the intestines.[165] The heart is the center of all solicitude and care: the lungs cool it should it flame up in wrath, and the lungs are the center of the vital spirit, or *pneuma*.[166] There are two channels (or chambers) in the heart, both of which contain blood, but the right one contains more of the vital spirit. The region near the heart is the precordium, and moves with the heartbeat and respirations.[167] The pulse can be simple or complex in its motion, the former being normal. When in good health, the pulse is regular—"dactylic"—but unusual rapidity, weakness, or irregularity is an important sign of illness. Like other ancients, Isidore does not distinguish between arteries and veins, but refers to channels which transport blood throughout the body for its nutrition. The quantity of blood diminishes in old age.[168]

The mechanical roles of the mouth, tongue, and teeth in eating are well and clearly described.[169] The throat, trachea and their relations are described, and the tonsils are mentioned with a remark on the frequency of enlarged tonsils. The hard and soft palates are distinguished, and their individual functions noted.[170] The mouth [171] is compared to the door of the belly which receives and passes on food to the intestines through the esophagus which is near the windpipe, and which is closed off by the epiglottis during deglutition.[172] The intestines are arranged in long circular entwinings so

[144] XI. 1. 32–36.
[145] XI. 1. 36–42.
[146] XI. 1. 22, 46.
[147] XI. 1. 22, 47–48.
[148] XI. 1. 51–53.
[149] XI. 1. 20–21.
[150] XI. 1. 23.
[151] XI. 1. 25.
[152] XI. 1. 86.
[152] XI. 1. 83–84.
[154] XI. 1. 88.
[155] XI. 1. 87.
[156] XI. 1. 95–96.
[157] XI. 1. 61, 95.
[158] XI. 1. 107.
[159] XI. 1. 111–115.

[160] XI. 1. 60.
[161] XI. 1. 60–71.
[162] XI. 1. 72–73.
[163] XI. 1. 89–93.
[164] XI. 1. 101.
[165] XI. 1. 116–117.
[166] XI. 1. 124.
[167] XI. 1. 118–119.
[168] XI. 1. 121–123.
[169] XI. 1. 49–51.
[170] XI. 1. 55–58.
[171] Or perhaps the stomach, since the text at this point is obscure; XI. 1. 128.
[172] XI. 1. 59.

that food can be gradually digested. The abdominal viscera are separated from the heart and lungs by the diaphragm and covered by the omentum.[173] Food, when first passed into the small intestine, is called *jantaculum*.[174] The large intestine, the "blind gut," is identified and it is pointed out that the gastrointestinal tract is open at each end.[175] The rectum and anus are turned away from our faces to spare us the indelicacy of witnessing their evacuation.[176]

The liver is the seat of elemental fire, whence it is diffused to the remainder of the body, and it is the liver which changes the juice obtained from the digestion of food into blood for bodily nutrition.[177] The spleen counterbalances the liver, an ancient idea, and is the seat of laughter. Gall is thought to be produced by and stored in the gallbladder.[178] Urine is collected from the kidneys: it sometimes burns when it is voided, and is carefully examined by the physician for signs of disease. The bladder is named as though it were a water vessel, and is distended by urine, but it does not have this function in birds.[179]

The skin not only protects the body against injury, but against rain, wind, and the sun's heat. Isidore points out that a subcutaneous muscular layer is found in animals but not in man. The pores are breathing holes, through which the vital spirit passes. The panniculus adiposus is identified.[180]

The Pythagorean view is taught that the male's semen comes from the kidneys, where it is formed by the repeated evaporation and condensation of a thinner liquid derived from the spinal cord and the other parts of the body.[181] It is supplied by the testes to the penis.[182] "The male's semen is the froth of blood shaken up like water on the rocks at the seashore, which makes the spume white, or as dark wine shaken in the cup turns white." [183] Isidore reports that eunuchs, while sometimes potent, are sterile:

Eunuch, *eunuchus*, is the Greek word which means "castrated." Some of these are able to have coitus, but there is no fertility in their semen. They have a fluid, and ejaculate it, but it is weak and useless for procreation.[184]

173 XI. 1. 129–130.
174 XX. 2. 10.
175 XI. 1. 131–132.
176 XI. 1. 105, 133.
177 XI. 1. 125.
178 XI. 1. 127–128.
179 XI. 1. 137–138.
180 XI. 1. 78–81.
181 XI. 1. 97, 139.
182 XI. 1. 102–103.
183 IX. 6. 4.
184 X. 93. Isidore attended the Second Council of Bracara, which ruled that a candidate for ordination, if his genitalia had been amputated by a physician on medical grounds, or by savages, might be ordained, but that if he had castrated himself, he could not be ordained. Self-castration after ordination disqualified him. The medical indications are not related. See *Concilium Bracarense II*, Chapter 21 [*PL* 84: 577–578].

Sexual desire has its beginnings in the loins in men and in the umbilicus in women.[185] The genitalia are the bodily parts of generation, often called the *pudenda* because of modesty, or because of the growth of hair which occurs there at puberty. Only men have a penis and the testes, "witnesses" to virility, are located in the "pouch." [186] The vulva is named by analogy to a folding door (*valva*): it receives the semen and discharges the fetus. Only women have a womb and its adnexa, shaped together like a ram's horn. The uterus is also called the *matrix*, since it shapes and forms the fetus through an admixture of semen with menstrual blood under the influence of the body's heat.[187]

Menstrual blood is a monthly flow: woman is the only menstrual animal.[188] At certain times, semen is not germinable because if no menstrual blood is present, pregnancy does not result, but the semen itself may be defective through excessive thickness or thinness.[189] Milk is produced in the breasts from blood not needed for intrauterine nourishment of the fetus after parturition: when the breasts swell up with milk, infants suck.[190] The infant is nourished in the womb through its umbilical cord.[191] The heart is the first part of the human body to be formed, and the fetus is completely shaped—as is learned from abortions—by the fortieth day after conception. In birds, the eyes develop first, as is learned from the examination of eggs. The fetus is surrounded by membranes which are delivered after it. The physical characteristics of children are determined by the relative strength of the male and female seeds required for each conception, and in the classical tradition, the child's sex is determined by the relative position of his parents at the time of impregnation.[192]

ISIDORE'S AGES OF MAN

Isidore divides the human lifespan into six stages: infancy, from birth until seven; childhood, which ends either at puberty or at fourteen; adolescence, from puberty until full maturity at twenty-eight; youth, which in the classical tradition lasts until fifty; maturity, which embraces the years between fifty and seventy—the individual is no longer young, but is not yet old; old age is whatever remains after the age of seventy, and senility is the extreme end of old age, ending in death.[193] Etymologies are provided for the names of these stages,[194] and the characteristics of each stage are explained in the light of the humoral pathology.[195] Old

185 XI. 1. 98.
186 XI. 1. 102–104.
187 XI. 1. 134–136, 139.
188 XI. 1. 140.
189 XI. 1. 142.
190 XI. 1. 75–77.
191 XI. 1. 99.
192 XI. 1. 143–145.
193 XI. 2. 1–8.
194 XI. 2. 9–18.
195 XI. 2. 27.

age has its compensations no less than its handicaps, but all things considered, it is a good stage of life, barring illness and extreme senility.[196] Death and funerary rites are discussed in their appropriate place following the discussion of senility.[197]

Isidore thinks that women are weaker than men physically but that this implies no defect in her composition, since this was intended by the Creator.[198] He notes that women's sexual passions are stronger than men's, and seems to imply that they increase with age.[199]

ISIDORE'S PORTENTOUS MONSTERS AND TRANSFORMATIONS

Chapter three of *Etymologiae* XI includes a study of monsters, beginning with a derivation of the word taken from Varro, and carefully qualified by the observation that a monster does not in any way arise contrary to nature but contrary to what we understand to be nature.[200] Many ancient writers believed that the birth of a monster portended some important future event, and, although Isidore cites examples of this, it is not always clear from his carefully qualified statements whether or not he actually believed or disbelieved in such prodigies.[201] There is a methodical discussion of just what makes a monster unusual: size and excess or defect of parts are the chief factors, although whole races are regarded as monsters.[202] His sources are chiefly classical mythology and the folklore of giants and pygmies, together with embellishments of the congenital anomalies of obstetric literature and those unfortunate creatures who in less sophisticated days were the attractions of circus sideshows.[203] There is a reference to a case attributed to Aristotle of *situs inversus viscerum*.[204] Among other monsters are cited such anomalies as polydactylism, oligodactylism, and hermaphroditism.[205]

Isidore's discussion of monsters, by which he means both the monsters of literature and the anomalies and malformations of medical practice, is rational and more than a little skeptical. The legend that the giants were born after the cohabitation of fallen angels with the daughters of men is mentioned only for condemnation.[206] Many monsters, chiefly from classical myths and ancient travelers' tales are treated as hearsay, or provided with rational explanations. Legends of childhood marriage in India have perhaps been transmuted into an account of a race in India whose women conceive at five and, possibly because of their fearful childbed mortality, do not live past the age of eight.[207] Many standard monsters of classical mythology—Gorgons, Scylla, Sirens, Cereberus, the Hydra—are described with a more natural explanation by treating these as allegories concealing an underlying factual event.[208]

Travel was difficult, expensive, and dangerous in Isidore's world, and any individual man's horizons were narrowly bounded. The blonde hair and blue eyes of the Angles astonished not only Caesar's armies but Gregory the Great, and it took more than one last battle to convince Roman legions that Britons could swim a river too deep to ford. Isidore's monsters are no medieval Madam Tussaud's of demonology but fall somewhere between a classical dictionary discussion of mythology and a primitive Gould's *Anomalies and Curiosities of Medicine*. In many cases, it is not difficult to ascribe factual origin to these monsters: remote, twisted, and exaggerated, but factual.

ISIDORE'S MEDICINE

Compared with the other books of the *Etymologiae*, Isidore's book on medicine is exceptionally brief and its definitions remarkably curt. It contains little on surgery and nothing on midwifery. His few observations on surgery are descriptive, and although amputation, cupping, and cauterization are mentioned, little detailed information is provided. The medical definitions are usually sufficiently complete to permit identification of the symptoms or processes which Isidore has in mind, and because ancient physicians did not have a coherent pathology or physiology, a symptom (e.g., jaundice) is often considered as though it were a disease. Isidore's medicine is derived entirely from books, and the standard medical writers of his time pay rather little attention to midwifery and surgery. Both of these crafts were (and, in large measure, are) learned by apprenticeship, and their practitioners were sometimes nearly or quite illiterate. Midwifery has only recently been practiced by physicians, and church authorities seem always to have discouraged priests from performing surgical operations, since a priest responsible for death following the spilling of blood incurs certain impediments to his ritual duties. It is most probable that *Etymologiae* IV was intended only to provide definitions of unfamiliar technical medical terms, and not as a manual of medical practice for beginners.

Isidore states that all diseases arise within the body from disharmony among the four humors, and that health consists in a proper balance among them. Effective treatment requires that a middle course be found between the disease process and what the body will tolerate,[209] since overtreatment and the habitual use of medicines are vexatious and fraught with danger.[210]

[196] XI. 2. 29–30.
[197] XI. 2. 31–37.
[198] XI. 2. 19–20.
[199] XI. 2. 24–25.
[200] XI. 3. 1–2.
[201] XI. 3. 3–5.
[202] XI. 3. 6–12.
[203] XI. 3. 13–14.
[204] XI. 3. 9.
[205] XI. 3. 7–11.
[206] XI. 3. 13.

[207] XI. 3. 27.
[208] XI. 3. 28–29.
[209] IV. 5. 2–3.
[210] IV. 2.

The acute diseases arise from an excess of blood or of yellow bile, chronic diseases from an excess of phlegm or black bile.[211] Acute diseases tend to death or recovery within a short time,[212] but the chronic diseases tend to a protracted course.[213] Nowhere does Isidore ascribe disease in human beings to direct supernatural intervention, although God may permit disease to serve His own purposes.[214] Special etiologies are given some diseases, over and above the humors: rabies comes from the bite of a mad dog, or from contact with its saliva.[215] Plague is an epidemic disease of sudden onset and rapid course spread by corrupt air: although these "air-borne potencies" penetrate the viscera to produce disease, a pestilence does not spread without the permission of Almighty God.[216] There is a detailed humoral explanation for the production of pus, and "bloody matter," probably pus in general, and "decomposition," probably wet gangrene and tissue necrosis—with their different prognoses—are defined.[217]

Isidore defines medicine in the Galenic tradition as the art which protects and preserves or restores bodily health, embracing not only the treatment of diseases and wounds, but diet and hygiene as well.[218] In this, he follows the late classical tradition, and derives the name of medicine from *modus,* perhaps best translated as "an observation of due proportion." [219]

This introduction is followed by the earliest medieval account of the history of medicine. Apollo is credited with the invention of medicine, which was augmented and improved upon by his "son," Aesculapius. The tradition of Aesculapius' death by lightning is recorded, and Hippocrates is named as the descendant of Aesculapius who restored the art of medicine.[220] Isidore mentions nothing of Prehippocratic medicine, but comments that, in more ancient times, medicine was based on the use of herbs and became more complex with time.[221] He comments on a kind of evolution in diet when he notes that before grain was cultivated, men lived on wild herbs and acorns.[222]

In the ancient tradition again, Isidore divides treatment into the three branches of pharmaceutical, surgical, and dietetic, the latter including hygiene and nursing arts.[223] He is emphatic when he insists that the resources of human medicine are not to be despised, and cites scriptural support for this position, perhaps to discourage undue reliance upon faith-healing, itself not

particularly prominent in the medical views of early churchmen.[224] There was apparently no little popular resort to magic rites and modes of treatment, denounced both by Isidore and the physicians of the time.[225] The three principal sects into which medicine split in postclassical times—Methodist, Logical or Dogmatic, and Empiric—are briefly discussed, with a special encomium for Hippocrates and the Logical sect, which had been represented by Cassius Felix. The later Pneumatic and Eclectic schools are not mentioned.[226] A discussion of the therapeutic use of "similars" and "contraries" suggests not only the possibility of an ancient allopathic-homeopathic controversy, but documents some confusion over the finer details of the humoral pathology, and the unsatisfactory state of the therapy at the time.[227] Isidore refers to the legend that Chiron developed veterinary medicine, and that it is for this reason that he is depicted as half-man and half-horse.[228] The semilegendary figure of Asclepiades is described as having cured an insane man through the use of music, which in ancient times included both the dance and eurhythmics, a reason why the physician ought to study music.[229]

Medical books mentioned in the discussion, although Isidore certainly knew of more, are the Hippocratic *Aphorisms* and *Prognostics,*[230] early known through Latin translations from the Greek. Two distinct kinds of herbal are mentioned: *Dinamidia,* which describe the actions of and indications for vegetable drugs, the use of animal and mineral products being relatively infrequent, and *Butanicum,* herbals which describe and illustrate the plants with medicinal value, such as the books mentioned by Cassiodorus.[231] Galen is cited by name as an authority in a discussion of the changes in innate heat which occur at the various ages of life, but the title of the work mentioned is so corrupt that it cannot be identified.[232]

In Isidore's discussion of disease, which is quite in accord with the views of other early Churchmen, there is remarkably little support for the notion that disease arises from specific sins or vices. He points out that physical infirmity arises from three causes: sin, temptation and intemperance of the bodily passions, and that, although human medicines are able to help the latter,

---

211 IV. 5. 7.
212 IV. 6. 1.
213 IV. 7. 1.
214 IV. 6. 17.
215 IV. 6. 15.
216 IV. 6. 17–19, see also Isidore, *De natura rerum* 39.
217 IV. 8. 22.
218 IV. 1. 1–2.
219 IV. 2.
220 IV. 3. 1–2; VIII. 11. 3; VIII. 11. 53.
221 IV. 9. 4.
222 XVII. 7. 26; XVII. 10. 2.
223 IV. 9. 2–3.

224 IV. 9. 1.
225 VIII. 9, passim.
226 IV. 4. 1–2.
227 IV. 9. 5–7.
228 IV. 13. 3.
229 IV. 9. 12.
230 IV. 10. 1–2.
231 IV. 10. 3–4; see Cassiodorus, *Institutiones* I. 21.
232 XX. 2. 37: "Physicians and those who have written on the nature of the human body, especially Galen in those books whose title is †PERSIE in quo†, say that the bodies of boys and young men, and of men and women of mature age, are warm with an internal heat, and that those foods are harmful at these ages which increase this heat, but that those things are healthy taken as food which tend to coolness just as, on the contrary, the elderly—who suffer from phlegm and cold—profit from heat-producing foods and ripe wines."

only Divine mercy avails the two former.[233] He suggests an overlapping difference between illness of the body, *aegrotatio*, and that of the soul, *aegritudo*, the former referring only to physical illness, the latter to subjective distress which apparently needs have no necessary relationship to physical factors.[234]

When discussing nervous and mental diseases, which he generally considers chronic, Isidore is as free from superstition as the medical writers of his day, and natural causes are consistently ascribed even these maladies. Epilepsy is discussed under various synonyms,[235] but Isidore is wrong when he reports that the quail (*ortygometra*) is the only animal other than man subject to epilepsy.[236] Isidore considers lunacy a form of epilepsy, not demonic possession,[237] and mania a disordered state of mind characterized by fury and agitation,[238] as distinguished from the depression which Isidore calls *melancholia*[239] to form a rough but realistic classification of psychiatric illness, depending upon domination of the clinical picture by disorientation, by hyperactivity, or by social withdrawal and feelings of mistrust. Isidore lists a number of drugs which induce mental changes: hellebore or veratrum,[240] mandrake, some species of which have an atropine effect,[241] opium,[242] henbane,[243] and coriander.[244]

Isidore regards masturbation only as an effeminate habit,[245] and *faute de mieux* male homosexuality is mentioned briefly in passing.[246] Senile dementia is thought to be a state of mind parallel to early childhood, mental weakness in the former state resulting from advanced years and in the latter from irresponsibility and lack of maturity.[247] Dementia and mental deficiency are distinguished.[248] Musical therapy is recommended for the mentally and emotionally upset, without reference to etiology or resort to violence or superstition.[249] During ancient times, epilepsy and mental disease generally were thought to be influenced by the moon's cycle, and Isidore shares this view.[250]

In the *Differentiarum*, Isidore is at some pains to define a few descriptive psychiatric terms. He notes the difference between a man who is drunk (*ebrius*) and a habitual drunkard (*ebriosus*): one drinks too much for a time, the other always drinks too much.[251] Likewise, he distinguishes between an insane man (*insanus*) and one enraged or blinded by passion (*insaniens*): one is in a state of permanent mental fury, the other is impelled by sudden wrath or indignation.[252] *Dementia* and *delirium* are distinguished, and although the demented (*demens*) individual can be of any age, Isidore seems to restrict *delirium* to something akin our concept of senile dementia, probably reserving *frenesis* for other types of delirium. He provides an etymology for *delirium*, relating it to inability to speak in an orderly fashion.[253] *Dementia* can be distinguished from *amentia*, only because the former is temporary or develops over a period of time, while the latter is permanent.[254]

Isidore has a low opinion of alcoholism: he mentions that, although overeating produces gluttonous surfeit, overindulgence in drink produces disturbances of the intellect, disordered emotions, and burning lust. He points out that the drunkard loses his intellect, may forget where he is or what evils he has committed, and reinforces this by some Old Testament

[233] Isidore, *Sententiarum* III. 3. 4 [*PL* 83: 658–659].
[234] Isidore, *Differentiarum* I. 69–70 [*PL* 83: 17–18].
[235] IV. 7. 5–7.
[236] XII. 7. 65.
[237] IV. 7. 6.
[238] IV. 7. 8.
[239] IV. 7. 9; X. 176.
[240] XVII. 9. 24: "Hellebore recalls a certain town in Greece in the vicinity of *Elleborum* where much of it grows and from which it is named by the Greeks. The Romans call this by another name, *veratrum*, since if it is taken, it leads a disturbed mind to health. There are two kinds: white and black."
Veratrum is still used in the treatment of hypertension, and relief of the mental symptoms of hypertensive encephalopathy can be dramatic.
[241] XVII. 9. 30: "Mandrake, *mandragora*, is so named because it has sweet-smelling fruit, about the size of a Matian apple; for this reason, the Latins call it the 'earth apple.' The poets call it 'man-shaped,' *ANTHROPOMORPHOS*, because it has a root shaped like a human figure. The root of this plant, mixed with wine, is given those people to drink whose bodies are to be operated upon in hope of curing them, so that under the influence of this soporific, they may not feel the pain. There are two species of this fruit: the female, which leaves shaped like those of lettuce, bearing plum-shaped fruit, and, on the other hand, the male, which has leaves like a beet."
[242] XVII. 9. 31: "The poppy is the sleep-bearing herb, of which Vergil says [*Georgics* 1. 78]: *Lethaeo perfusa papavera somno*, 'Heavy sleep, pressed out of the poppy,' since it stupefies the sleeper. Some poppies are common; others are stronger, namely those from which flows the juice called *opion*."
[243] XVII. 9. 41: "Henbane, *hyoscyamos*, is named from the Greek, and is called 'the calicular herb' by the Latins because it grows little cups shaped like tankards, like those of the pomegranate, whose edges are serrated, having seeds inside similar to those of the poppy. This herb is also called 'unhealthy,' *insana*, because its use is so dangerous, for it happens that if it be eaten or drunk, it produces insanity or clouding of the mind similar to sleep. The common people call this insanity *milimindrum*, because it induces alienation of mind."
[244] XVII. 11. 7.
[245] X. 179.
[246] XI. 2. 19.
[247] XI. 2. 27.
[248] X. 79.
[249] IV. 13. 3; III. 17. 3; III. 22. 1, 6.
[250] IV. 7. 6.
[251] Isidore, *Differentiarum* I. 205 [*PL* 83: 31].
[252] Isidore, *Differentiarum* I. 297 [*PL* 83: 40].
[253] Isidore, *Differentiarum* I. 140 [*PL* 83: 25]: "Demens est cujuscunque aetatis amens, et sine mente, delirus autem per aetatem mente defectus: dictus autem ita, eo quod recto ordine, quasi lira, aberret. Lira enim est orationis genus, cum agricola facta, semente dirigunt sulcos."
Cf. below, IV. 7. 8. Souter defines *liro*, "be out of one's mind."
[254] Isidore, *Differentiarum* I. 144 [*PL* 83: 25]; see below, IV. 7. 8 and XI. 1. 13.

condemnations of drunkenness.[255] He notes the rapidity with which it produces hyperemia in his derivation of the word "wine." [256]

Isidore's neurology is entirely descriptive: *frenesis* is apparently any disease characterized by agitation and dementia, so that this could apply equally well to delirium tremens or to acute meningoencephalitis.[257] Headache is a chronic disease, but ancient writers often refer to the protracted dull headache of malaria, and this may be meant.[258] Scotoma is differentiated from vertigo, which is given a humoral explanation.[259] "Lethargy" seems to include stupor and coma from any cause, and the snoring respiration of a deeply unresponsive patient with a central nervous system insult is carefully described.[260] Apoplexy is correctly ascribed to a sudden hemorrhage.[261] Muscular spasm and the opisthotonos of meningeal irritation are both described, and given etymologies.[262] Sciatica is thought to arise from a condensation of phlegm in the long bones of the thighs, an etiology perhaps explicable in terms of symptomatic relief from dry heat.[263] Paralysis may result in one part of the body appearing cooler than the remainder.[264] The two forms of nyctalopia, day blindness and night blindness, are carefully distinguished.[265]

In what is called "cardiac disease," there is sharp pain of the region of the anterior chest and upper abdomen accompanied by extreme apprehension: this refers to almost any pain of the mediastinal and epigastric region, and Isidore's definition is not limited to the heart.[266] Pleurisy is a sharp pain in the side accompanied by fever and a bloody sputum.[267] Pneumonia is accompanied by a sighing respiration, and Isidore lists it with both the acute and chronic diseases, retaining the same word (*peripleumonia*) for a swelling of the lung accompanied by bloody sputum.[268] Cough and hemoptysis are mentioned only as symptoms.[269] Phthisis is a chronic disease especially common in young people, and is marked by a gradual wasting of the whole body.[270] It is doubtful that pulmonary neoplasm was very often distinguished from pulmonary tuberculosis in ancient times on clinical grounds. Empyema is described in general terms as an internal abscess.[271] Dropsy is a subcutaneous collection of fluid, but Isidore does not repeat the classical division of dropsy into ascites, anasarca and edema.[272]

Laryngitis and bronchitis are merely mentioned as causes of hoarseness,[273] but *synanche,* a swelling and constriction of the throat, can lead to death by suffocation.[274] Coryza, the common cold, is merely an annoying nasal discharge accompanied by sneezing.[275] Asthma is correctly attributed to respiratory constriction with resulting dyspnea.[276] Recurrent fevers perhaps of undulant and malarial types are mentioned, but their description is too meagre to permit identification if, indeed, they still occur.[277] Fevers generally stem from an overabundance of heat.[278]

Gastritis may refer only to the pain of gastric irritation, but since described as associated with fever, the possibility of a perforated or at least active gastric ulcer must be considered.[279] Colic, according to Isidore's brief description, refers to abdominal pain in general, and cannot be interpreted as anything more specific than that group of disorders which surgeons now describe as an "acute abdomen," whether due to perforation of a viscus, strangulation of a hernia, or something else seriously amiss within the abdomen.[280] Hepatic and splenic disease are merely defined as affections of the organs in question,[281] and *nefresis* is thought to be a weakness of the kidneys.[282]

Cachexia can be part of a long convalescence from disease, or the result of the patient's indiscretion or the physician's mismanagement. Atrophy is a localized wasting which is the result of cessation of nourishment to the part affected.[283] *Sarcia* may be merely obesity, but, although some manuscripts read *sarcoma,* a local tumor probably is not intended.[284] Diarrhea and dysentery are distinguished, and a condition which suggests sprue or celiac disease is described.[285] Gout is characterized by its beastly pain, and differs from arthritis, which is a simple disease of the joints.[286] Vesical calculus, strangury, and priapism are very briefly defined.[287]

Carbuncle, stye, and abscess are defined,[288] and

[255] Isidore, *Sententiarum* II. 43. 1–2 [*PL* 83: 649–650] and XX. 2. 9.
[256] XX. 3. 2: "Wine is so named because its drinking quickly fills the veins with blood."
[257] IV. 6. 3.
[258] IV. 7. 2.
[259] IV. 7. 3–4.
[260] IV. 6. 5.
[261] IV. 6. 10.
[262] IV. 6. 11–13.
[263] IV. 7. 29.
[264] IV. 7. 25.
[265] IV. 8. 8.
[266] IV. 6. 4.
[267] IV. 6. 8.
[268] IV. 6. 9; IV. 7. 15.
[269] IV. 7. 16, 18.
[270] IV. 7. 17.

[271] IV. 7. 20.
[272] IV. 7. 23.
[273] IV. 7. 14.
[274] IV. 6. 6.
[275] IV. 7. 11–12.
[276] IV. 7. 14.
[277] IV. 7. 10.
[278] IV. 6. 2.
[279] IV. 6. 7.
[280] IV. 7. 14, 38.
[281] IV. 7. 21–22.
[282] IV. 7. 24.
[283] IV. 7. 26–27.
[284] IV. 7. 28.
[285] IV. 7. 35–38.
[286] IV. 7. 30–31.
[287] IV. 7. 32–34.
[288] IV. 8. 15–16.

there is an important distinction between ulcers and wounds: ulcers are a breach in the skin of endogenous origin, not directly related to trauma; wounds are the result of external force or violence.[289] Alopecia is mentioned, but Isidore's description apparently refers to a chronic infection accompanied by loss of hair rather than to ordinary baldness.[290] Parotitis is a firm swelling or abscess near the ears following a fever, and may thus refer to endemic mumps or to bacterial infection.[291] Erysipelas, herpes, and impetigo are accurately described.[292] There is a differential diagnosis betwen scabies and leprosy apparently derived from Leviticus.[293] Common warts and pityriasis are distinguished.[294] Pruritis[295] and jaundice[296] are defined, and the latter is considered only as a disease of the skin, for which a full diet is indicated. Pustules and papules are described in very modern terms.[297]

There is a reference to an elephantiasis which seems to be a chronic indurated skin infection or cellulitis, perhaps a form of scleroderma, rather than brawny lymphedema.[298] The patient with cancer, although his illness is incurable, may live longer if a palliative amputation is performed, since drugs are ineffective.[299] Perioral ulcers which occur in adults and children are described: these may be the result of vitamin deficiency or be aphthous stomatitis.[300] Fistulae are only mentioned by name without description.[301] Isidore seems to use the word *cicatrix* for both the granulation tissue in a wound which is healing by secondary or tertiary intention, and for the formed scar which results.[302] Rhagades and hemorrhoids are confused, but the latter are correctly described.[303]

Many plants were listed in ancient herbals and books on materia medica, and Isidore includes most of the ancient vegetable drugs with predictable effects in his seventeenth book, "On agriculture." Omitting a formidable list ascribed curious functions in folklore and overlooking those "said to arouse venery," some of these plants are still in use. Thyme was a diuretic and emmenagogue,[304] the citron an antidote for serpent venom,[305] and the prune highly thought of as a food for stomach disorders which were often aggravated

by other fruits.[306] Elderly people ate figs to smooth out their wrinkles.[307] Willow seeds taken in wine increased love for children but made women infertile.[308] An unidentifiable herb, *amomum,* produces deep sleep,[309] and hyacinth roots kept boys from reaching puberty.[310]

Two kinds of veratrum, or hellebore, are identified, useful in leading the mentally disturbed to health.[311] Euphorbium was highly regarded as an eyewash and as an emollient for indurated wounds.[312] Assafoedita is mentioned without directions for its use.[313] An ointment made from dittany was the usual topical application for injuries incurred in war.[314] Mandrake root is described without reference to folklore, and directions are given for steeping it in wine to prepare a soporific for those about to undergo surgical operations.[315] Two species of poppy are described, from one of which opium is prepared, and, although directions are provided for its preparation, its use is not mentioned in detail.[316] Warts were removed by heliotrope tea or poultices or heliotrope leaves applied locally.[317] Hyssop is an expectorant.[318] Henbane, or hyoscine, apparently had serious side effects including a specific form of insanity.[319] *Saxifraga* was

[289] IV. 8. 19.
[290] IV. 8. 1.
[291] IV. 8. 2.
[252] IV. 8. 4–6.
[293] IV. 8. 10–11; see Leviticus 13. 1–6.
[294] IV. 8. 9.
[295] IV. 8. 7.
[256] IV. 8. 13.
[297] IV. 8. 20–21.
[2ዐ8] IV. 8. 12.
[299] IV. 8. 14.
[300] IV. 8. 17.
[301] IV. 8. 22.
[302] IV. 8. 23.
[303] IV. 8. 39.
[304] IV. 12. 2; XVII. 9. 51 refers to thyme's emmenagogue reputation.
[305] XVII. 7. 8.

[306] XVII. 7. 10: ". . . This is the only fruit proved to remedy the stomach, for other fruits are said to be harmful. Only this tree distills a gum which is gluey and suitable for joining, used both by physicians and writers."
[307] XVII. 7. 17: "The fig, *ficus,* is named from fecundity, since it is more fruitful than other trees. It bears fruit three or four times in a single year, and as one crop is ripening, another springs up. Hence also it is named *carica* because of its copiousness, *copia.* It is said that the Egyptian fig is more fecund, the wood of which, being thrust into water and left for a little while in a marshy place, if the part growing above the ground be taken away, contrary to the force of nature, it will remain soaked by a large remaining quantity of water. Formerly athletes were fed on figs before the trainer Pythagoras changed them over to the use of flesh meat, which is a more nourishing food. Figs are often taken by the elderly in their food because they are said to smooth out their wrinkles. It is also said that fierce bulls tethered to a fig-tree suddenly become quieter."
[308] XVII. 7. 47.
[309] XVII. 8. 11.
[310] XVII. 9. 15.
[311] XVII. 9. 24, and see note 240 above.
[312] XVII. 9. 26: "*Euphorbium* is so named because its juice improves the vision. Its power is such that if it is applied to fleshy indurations, it quickly forces them to soften. It grows in many places, but most abundantly in Mauretania."
[313] XVII. 9. 27.
[314] XVII. 9. 29: "*Dicta* is a mountain in Crete, from which the herb takes the name *dictamnum,* dittany, in search of which in Vergil [*Aeneid* 4. 73], the wounded hind wandered through the Dictaean woodlands. This has such power that it can expel iron weapons from the body and remove arrows; whence it is that wild beasts that have eaten it, struck by arrows, cast off those adhering to their bodies. Some of the Latins call this the 'fleabane of Mars,' *puleium Martis,* because of its usefulness in extracting arrows during war."
[315] XVII. 9. 30, and see note 241 above.
[316] IV. 9. 8; XVII. 9. 31 and see note 242 above.
[317] XVII. 9. 36.
[318] XVII. 9. 39.
[319] XVII. 9. 41, and see note 243 above.

thought to be able to reduce and break up bladder stones.[320] Gentian, the orchid, cole-wart, and coriander were credited with aphrodisiac power,[321] among many other things, but sorrel was not only an antiaphrodisiac which calmed the fires of lust, but strengthened the stomach withal.[322] Caperspurge was a rapidly acting cathartic,[323] but hemlock is recalled only for its role in the execution of Socrates.[324] Nightshade, or strychnine, was used for headache and stomach pain.[325] Anise was another diuretic,[326] and mulberry juice was used for a wide variety of ills.[327]

There are few details about nonvegetable drugs: Samian earth is mentioned as used by physicians, but just how is not stated.[328] Sulfur[329] and niter[330] are also noted but also lack specific details. Common salt is described as astringent and drying to the skin.[331] Cantharides, "Spanish fly," is described only as a powerful vesicant, and is assigned no aphrodisiac effects.[332]

Isidore lists a wide variety of incenses, perfumed medicinal oils, plasters, salves, cathartics, expectorants, serpent antivena, electuaries, lozenges, and eye-salves and washes. Wound compresses, poultices, plasters, enemata both cleansing and medicated and pessaries, which were not limited to gynecological practice but included medications inserted into any bodily orifice, complete the list of therapeutic equipment, although little detailed information is provided as to their composition or use.[333]

Surgical instruments include the bistoury,[334] various probes and sounds, the sharp hooks used in ancient times as forceps,[335] cupping instruments, syringes of various sizes and uses, what seems to be an eyecup, mortars and pestles, and,[336] of course, an instrument case.[337] The cautery is described with both factual medical and allegoric moral etymologies.[338] Poultices

and plasters of various sorts were applied, but specific surgical operations other than palliative amputation for cancer,[339] are not mentioned. For Isidore, circumcision is not a surgical operation, but a mark of membership in the Jewish race.[340] He knows about but does not describe infibulation.[341]

Isidore devotes some attention to parasitology, mentioning the round worm, the ascaris, the louse, its nits and the flea. He refers to a bacon worm, dog ear mites and bot flies.[342] His account of the leech and remarks as to how it gets into the human body is exact, but he mentions no medicinal use for leeches.[343] Serpent venom is considered at some length: the hemolytic effect of asp venom is described, and the account of viper venom is complete with a description of the snake's habits and the clinical course of a patient following envenomation.[344]

What is sometimes used as a mark of ownership, sometimes is applied as a cure, so that the power of disease may be dried up by the heat of fire."

[339] IV. 8. 14.
[340] XIX. 23. 7.
[341] XIX. 33. 4.
[342] XII. 5. 12–17: "Insects found in the flesh are: hemicranius; the round worm, lumbricus; ascaris, ascarida; bot fly, costus; louse, pediculus; flea, pulex; nits, lendes; bacon worm, tarmus; tick, ricinus; usia and bug, cimex. An insect infesting the head is hemicranius. Lumbricus is a worm in the intestines, so named from the haunch, lumbricus, because it glides along, labier; or because it is found in the loins. Ascaridae [. . .] Costi [. . .] Lice, pediculus, are insects inhabiting the skin, named after their feet, pes, whence people are termed 'lousy,' pediculosus, on whose bodies lice grow. The flea, pulex, is so named because it is especially to be found growing in dust, pulvis. Nits, lendes [. . .] Bacon-worm, tarmus, is a worm found in bacon. The tick, ricinus, is a worm infesting dogs, since it adheres in their ears: KUŌN is Greek for 'dog.' Usia is a worm of pigs, so called because it burns, and wherever it bites, itching and vesicles appear."
Probably 'bot-fly' is a fair translation for costus since the larval stage of the bot-fly causes horses to start and become difficult to manage because of their pain, although the stable fly (Stomoxys calcitrans) or gadfly (Tabnus septentrionalis) may be meant instead of the bot-fly (any one of a variety of Gastrophilus). Usia, as a parasite of swine, is hard to identify: warble flies, as grubs, can produce an itching vesicular reaction when burrowing in the skin, but usia may refer to the sarcoptic mange so common in swine, and any of the mange mites (Sarcoptes and Psoroptes) which bite and burrow may be intended.
[343] XII. 5. 3: "The leech, sanguisuga, is an aquatic worm so named because it sucks blood. It conceals itself in drinking water, and when it reaches the cheeks or somewhere else, it adheres, and sucks blood. When distended with blood over its capacity, it vomits what it has drunk, and again sucks fresher."
[344] Isidore discusses serpent venom at some length. XII. 4. 15: "The asp, aspis, is called haemorrhois because if anyone has been bitten by one, he sweats blood as though the veins had been dissolved and whatever was vital had poured out through the blood. The Greeks call 'blood,' HAIMA."
XII. 4. 39–42: "All serpents are cool by their natures, nor do they strike except when they grow heated. When they are cool, they touch nothing, whence it is also that their venom is more harmful during the day than at night. They are torpid during the coldness of night, and understandably, since they

[320] XVII. 9. 42.
[321] XVII. 9. 42, 43; XVII. 10.21; XVII. 11. 7.
[322] XVII. 10. 20.
[323] XVII. 9. 65.
[324] XVII. 9. 71.
[325] XVII. 9. 78.
[326] XVII. 11. 6.
[327] IV. 9. 8.
[328] XVI. 1. 7.
[329] XVI. 1. 9–10.
[330] XVI. 2. 7: "Niter, nitrum, derives its name from a place, for it is found in a town or region of Egypt, Nitria. Medicines are prepared from and soiled bodies and clothing cleaned with it. The nature of this is not much different from that of salt: it has the virtue of salt, and likewise is found dried and glistening on the seashore."
[331] XVI. 2. 6.
[332] XII. 5. 5.
[333] IV. 9. 8–11.
[334] IV. 11. 2.
[335] IV. 9. 3–4.
[336] IV. 9. 3–7, 11.
[337] IV. 11. 1.
[338] XX. 16. 8: "The cautery, cauterium, is named as though a 'cautionary burning,' cauturium, because it burns so that it may be a warning against anyone and a severe caution whose [property] it is when it is seen, so that avarice may be bridled.

Although some early medieval churchmen practiced as physicians, there is no evidence that Isidore did so, or even that he was particularly interested in medicine. For him, like grammar, it existed and deserved study. He thought very highly of medicine, and concludes his book with the observation, "Hence it is that medi-

are made cold by the night's dew. The force of coldness and baneful chills draw up into themselves the vapor of the body, whence also they twist themselves up into knots during the winter, but uncoil during the summer. Hence, whenever anyone is struck by the venom of serpents, first he becomes senseless, and afterwards, when that poison, *virus,* is warmed in him, it becomes heated and immediately kills the man. It is named venom, *venenum,* because it goes through the veins, and the diffusion of its poison through the veins disrupts the prosperous growth of the body and extinguishes life. But the venom is not able to cause harm unless it comes into contact with a man's blood. Lucan [9. 614]: *Noxia serpentium est admixto sanguine pestis,* 'The harmfulness of serpents is in the mixing of venom with blood.' All venom, however, has a cold nature, and from this cold venom the soul, whose nature is fire, flees."

Most snake vena toxic for man produce hemolysis, intravascular thrombosis and marked neuromuscular disturbances—Isidore's bloody sweat and insensibility.

cine is called a second philosophy, for each discipline claims the whole of man for itself. Just as by philosophy the soul, so also by medicine the body is healed." [345]

Without the cultivation of medicine and without the preservation and occasional amplification of the Latin medical vocabulary, it is doubtful that Greco-Roman medicine would have been a heritage for the medieval universities, and to which the contributions of the Arabs and of the classical Renaissance could add. This tradition of classical medicine as an intellectual discipline, with a precise vocabulary understood all over the western world and its firm conception of disease as a natural process which admitted of study and, sometimes, of therapeutic modification survived and was a part—even if only a part—of the foundation upon which the Renaissance physicians could build. The diligent and painstaking efforts of just such early medieval men as Isidore ought not be forgotten in the glory of Vesalius and Harvey.

[345] IV. 13. 5.

ISIDORE OF SEVILLE ON MAN AND MONSTERS

A translation of

ISIDORI ETYMOLOGIARUM SIVE ORIGINUM LIBER XI:

De Homine et Portentis

1. MAN AND HIS PARTS

1. Nature, *natura*, is named after that which brings anything to birth, for it is the power of making and of begetting. Some have said that this is God, by Whom all things are created and exist.

2. *Genus* is named from "to generate," *gigni*, the name for which is derived from the earth, from which all things spring up; for the earth is called *GÊ* in Greek.

3. Life, *vita*, is named because of vigor, or because it holds the power of being born and of increasing. Whence also trees are said to have life, because they spring up and grow.

4. Man, *homo*, is so called because he was made from the soil, *humus*, as is [also] said in Genesis [2: 7]: *Et creavit Deus hominem de humo terrae*, "And God created man from the dust of the earth." By an improper usage, however, it is announced that the whole man [was made] from two substances, that is, from the union of body and soul. For properly "man," *homo*, is from "soil," *humus*.

5. The Greeks however have called man *ANTHRO-POS* because he looks upward, having been raised from the soil to contemplate his Maker. This is what the poet Ovid means when he says [*Metamorphoses* 1. 84]:

> *Pronaque cum spectant animalia cetera terram,*
> *os homini sublime dedit caelumque videre*
> *iussit, et erectos ad sidera tollere vultus.*

"Whilst other animals look upon the earth with faces bent down, he gave to man an upright countenance and commanded him to look at heaven and to raise his face to the stars." Man, therefore, standing upright, looks upon the sky that he may seek God, not upon the earth as do beasts fashioned by nature with heads looking downward and subservient to their bellies.

6. Man is, however, double: interior and exterior. The interior man is the soul [and] the exterior man is the body.

7. The soul, *anima*, was so called by the pagans because they took it to be wind. Whence also "wind" is *ANEMOS* in Greek, because we seem to live by taking in air with our mouths, but this is most clearly false since the soul arises long before air can be taken in by the mouth, and is already alive in its mother's womb.

8. The soul, therefore, is not air as some who were not able to comprehend its incorporeal nature have thought.

9. The "vital spirit," *spiritus*, is the same as the soul of which the Evangelist speaks, saying [John 10: 18]: *Potestatem habeo ponendi animam meam, et rursus potestatem habeo sumendi eam*, "I have the power to lay down my spirit, and again I have the power of picking it up." Likewise, it is of this very soul of Our Lord that the aforesaid Evangelist speaks at the time of His passion, when he says [John 19: 30]: *Et inclinato capite emisit spiritum*, "And bowing His head he gave up His spirit." For what is it to give up the spirit if not to lay down [one's] soul?

10. But the soul is so named because it lives; the spirit is named either because of its spiritual nature, or because it imparts breath in the body.

11. Likewise, the mind, *animus*, is the same as the soul, but the soul pertains to life, the mind to deliberation. For this reason, philosophers say that life remains even without the mind, and the soul persists without the intellect: whence also the "mindless." For it is called the intellect that it may know; the mind, that it may will.

---

1. 1: This view of nature was a commonplace of ancient cosmology; see Servius *Georgics* 2. 49, and Lactantius, *Institutes* 2. 8. 21 [*CSEL* 19: 134].

1. 3: See Servius *Aeneid* 5. 81.

1. 4: Jacques Fontaine, *Isidore de Séville et la culture classique dans l'espagne wisigothique* (Paris, 1959), pp. 661–662, discusses the *homo ex humo* hypothesis, and see also Isidore, *Differentiarum* II. 47 [*PL* 83: 77] *and* II. 43 [*PL* 83: 76–77].

1. 5: An argument for some kind of human superiority derived from an erect posture seems to have been popular; see Sallust, *De conjuratione Catilinae* 1 and Isidore, *Differentiarum* II. 50 [*PL* 83: 78].

1. 11: In this translation, whenever possible—although neither Isidore nor other writers of his age were perfectly consistent, and the terms seem to have been sometimes very vaguely used—*mens* is translated as "intellect," *animus* as "mind," *anima* as "soul," and *spiritus* as "breath" or "vital spirit," depending on the context. Cf. Evelyn Underhill, *Mysticism: a study in the nature and development of man's spiritual consciousness* (New York, 1955), p. x: ". . . a genuine two-foldness in human nature—the difference in kind between *Animus* the surface-self and *Anima* the transcendental self, in touch with supernatural realities." Fontaine, *op cit.*, pp. 686–692, has a long discussion of this problem in Isidore's works. See also Servius *Aeneid* 10. 487; Lactantius, *De opificio Dei* 18. 3 [*CSEL* 27: 57] and Isidore, *Differentiarum* II. 94–97 [*PL* 83: 84].

12. The intellect, *mens,* is named because it is eminent in the soul, or because it remembers, *memini.* Whence also the forgetful are "mindless." Nor is it the soul but what is most excellent in the soul, as though its head or eye, which is called the mind. Whence also man himself is said to be an image of God because of his mind. However, all these [faculties] are joined to the soul so that it is a single thing, but diverse names are applied to the soul according to its different functions.

13. The memory, *memoria,* is also the intellect and for this reason those who are forgetful are "mindless." When it gives life to the body, it is the soul, *anima;* when it wills, it is the mind, *animus;* when it knows, it is the intellect, *mens;* when it remembers, it is the memory; when it judges correctly, it is the reason, *ratio;* when it breathes, it is the vital spirit, *spiritus;* when it perceives anything, it is called sensation, *sensus.* For the mind is called "sense" after the things which it senses, and "sentiment," *sententia,* is similarly derived.

14. The body, *corpus,* is named because, being corruptible, it perishes; for it is soluble and mortal, and some time will be dissolved.

15. But flesh, *caro,* is named from "creation," *creare.* There is power of increase in the male's semen from which the bodies of animals and men are conceived. Hence also, parents are called "creators."

16. The flesh, however, is composed of four elements: earth is in the fleshy parts, air in the breath, water in the blood, fire in the vital heat. For the elements each have in us a proper proportion, of which something is lacking when the conjunction is dissolved.

17. But "flesh," *caro,* and "body," *corpus,* indicate different things. The body is always in flesh, but flesh is not always in a body. For the flesh is that which lives, the same as a body. A body which is not alive is not the same thing as flesh, for it is possible to speak of a body either for that which, after life, is dead or that which was created lifeless. Sometimes a body can have life and yet be without flesh, as herbs and trees.

18. The bodily senses are five in number: sight, hearing, smell, taste and touch. Of these, two can be opened and closed off, while two are always open to sensation.

19. The senses are so called because through their agency the soul most acutely stirs the whole body with the force of perception. Whence "things present," *praesentia,* are so called because they are before, *prae,* the senses, as things which are at hand to the eyes are before the eyes.

20. Sight, *visus,* is located in what the philosophers call the *humor vitreus.* Some people affirm that seeing takes place either by an external ethereal light or an internal lucid spirit which come through delicate passages from the brain and after they have penetrated the coats of the eyes, come out into the air where they then give sight, being mixed with other similar matter.

21. Sight is so called because it is more vigorous than the other senses and is superior, or faster, and flourishes more fully even as memory [does] among the other faculties of the mind. It is closer to the brain, whence all things proceed, and for this reason, we refer things which properly pertain to the other senses to sight; as when we say "see" as in "see how it sounds," "see how it tastes" and other such things.

22. Hearing, *auditus,* is so called because it hears voices, that is, it takes up sounds from beaten air, *aër verberatus.* Smell, *odoratus,* is—so to speak—the touch of odor-bearing air. It is perceived by the air's touch. Smelling is the same thing, for it is caused by odors. Taste, *gustus,* is named after the gullet.

---

1. 12: The faculties of the soul are merely names applied to the soul's various functions; see Tertullian, *De anima* 14. 3 [Waszink 18] and Lactantius, *De opificio Dei* 16 [*CSEL* 27: 53].

1. 13: This passage defines the names applied to the faculties of the soul. One wonders how much of this equation of forgetfulness with "mindlessness" is a pedagogic trick. At *Differentiarum* II. 86 [*PL* 83: 82–83], Isidore differentiates between intelligence, *mens,* and reason, *ratio,* which he considers the application of the mind to the separation of truth from falsehood; and see also Servius Daniel *Aeneid* 2. 244.

1. 14: *Cf.* Tertullian, *De anima* 14. 1 [Waszink 17]: *nam et dividi dissolvi est et dissolvi mori est.*

1. 15: The definition of *carnes* is repeated at XX. 2. 20 in the context of food.

1. 16: This brief discussion of the four elements is developed in fuller detail at *Differentiarum* II. 48–49 [*PL* 83: 77–78], see pp. 23–25 above. There are other discussions of the elemental theory at, e.g., Lactantius, *Institutes* 2. 12. 12 [*CSEL* 19: 157] and Ambrose, *Hexameron* 1. 20 [*CSEL* 32: 17].

1. 17: Isidore amplifies this distinction between *flesh* and *body* at *Differentiarum* II. 93 [*PL* 83: 93].

1. 19: The ancients distinguished between a mental image and a visual hallucination; Lactantius, *De opificio Dei* 9 [*CSEL* 27: 31–32] has an involved discussion of diplopia, and Isidore, *Differentiarum* I. 216 [*PL* 83: 32] discusses phantasy and phantasms—the former depend on recollection of actual events and objects, the latter upon the imagination only. Nightmares are discussed at *Sententiarum* III. 6. 1–6 [*PL* 83: 668–669].

1. 20: Some of the vulgate manuscripts read *per tenues venas* instead of *per tenues vias.* Isidore discusses vision in much the same manner at *Sententiarum* I. 13. 3–4 [*PL* 83: 564], and see Lactantius, *De opificio Dei* 8 [*CSEL* 27: 31].

1. 21: See Varro, *De lingua latina* 6. 80.

1. 22: Alcmaeon of Croton (*fl. ca.* 500 B.C.) taught that hearing resulted from the concave shape of the middle ear, since hollow passages resound when noise enters them, and that odor was produced by the passage of odor-bearing elements through the nose to the brain. Ambrose, *Hexameron* 6. 63 [*CSEL* 32: 253] also distinguishes the sense of smell from odor as such, and *cf.* Isidore, III. 20. 2: "The voice is air set in motion [*lit.* 'beaten,' *verberatus*] by the breath."

23. Touch, *tactus*, is so called because it handles, feels, and spreads the force of sensation through all the members. We examine by touch whatever we cannot judge by the other senses. There are two kinds of touch: for either that which strikes comes from outside, or it arises within the body itself.

24. Every sense has been given its own proper nature: what is visible is apprehended by the eyes, what is audible by the ears; softness and hardness are evaluated by the touch; flavor by the taste, and odor by the nostrils.

25. The most important part of the body is the head, *caput:* it has been given this name because all sensation and nerves take their beginning thence, and because every principle of life springs therefrom. All of the senses are centered there and, in a certain manner, it plays the part of the soul itself which takes thought for the body.

26. The crown, *vertex*, is that part of the head where the hairs are gathered and around which the hairs are parted: hence its name.

27. The skull, *calvaria*, is named after the "bald bones," *ossa calva*, by ellipsis, and is inflected as a neuter. The occiput, *obcipitium*, is the posterior part of the head, as though it were opposite the head's covering, *capitium*, or as though it were "behind the head."

28. The hair, *capilli*, is named as though "the hairs of the head," *capitis pili*, created to add comeliness, to defend the brain against cold and to protect it from the sun. The hair, *pilus*, is named from the pelt, *pellis*, out of which it grows, just as the pestle, *pilum*, is named after the mortar, *pila*, in which drugs are ground up.

29. A head of hair, *caesaries*, is named from "cutting off," *caedere*, but this is true only of men. Cutting the hair is appropriate for men but not for women.

30. Hair, *coma*, is properly speaking "uncut hair," *non caesi capilli*, as it is in the Greek language, for the Greeks call the hair *caimos*, from "cutting off," whence also [they say] *KEIREIN*, "to cut off." And so, ringlets, *cirri*, which the Greeks call *MALLOS*, are named: curls, *crines*, refer to a coiffure proper to matrons.

31. Curls are also given that name because they are separated by ribbons: the things by which parted curls are bound are called hairpins, *discriminalis*.

32. The temples, *tempora*, lie to the left and right below the calvarium. They are so named because they are changed, and they are changed after certain intervals of time by that very mobility, just as the seasons.

33. The face, *facies*, is named from "likeness," *effigies*, since this reflects a man's whole personality and displays each individual's character.

34. The countenance, *vultus*, however, is so named because the soul's desires are shown by it, and it is changed according to the will, *voluntas*, into various motions; that is why they differ from each other. *Facies* simply signifies each one's natural appearance, but the countenance represents what sort of disposition he possesses.

35. The forehead, *frons*, is named from the apertures, *foramen*, for the eyes. This forms an image of the mind and expresses in its own way the motion of the intellect, whether it be happy or sad.

36. The eyes, *oculus*, are so called either because the roofs of the eyelids hide them, *occulare*, lest they be injured by something touching them, or because they contain some hidden, *occultus*, light, that is, secret or placed deep within. Among all the senses, these are thought to be the closest neighbors of the soul, and every disposition of the intellect is reflected in the eyes, whence also disturbance or hilarity of soul manifests itself in the eyes. But the eyes are also the same as "lamps," *lumina*, and they are called "lamps" because light, *lumen*, shines forth from them, or because from the very beginning they hold the light closed up within themselves, or because they reflect light received from outside to produce vision.

37. The pupil, *pupilla*, is the spot in the middle of the eye in which is located the power of seeing: because small images are apparent to us at this spot, they are called "pupils," Little boys are said to be "darlings," *pupillus*. Many even call this spot the "little girl," *pupula*: the pupil, *pupilla*, is called this because, like the little girls, it is pure and undefiled. Physicians say that those who are about to die do not have these little images which we see in the eyes for three days before death—it is certainly a desperate situation when these are not apparent.

38. The circle by which the white parts of the eye are separated from the pupil, marked by a distinct black color, is called the *corona*, because by its own roundness it embellishes the pupil's circumference.

39. The eyelids, *palpebrae*, form a bay for the eyes, and are named from their winking, *palpitare*, since

---

1. 25: Ambrose has a long teleological discussion of the head as the center of ·wisdom at *Hexameron* 6. 55–61 [*CSEL* 32: 251–252].

1. 27: *Calvarium* here is neuter, but is incorrectly given as feminine at XI. 1. 32; *calvaria, -ae*, also means "skull."

1. 30: Special coiffures were worn by married women and widows to distinguish them from unmarried women.

1. 32: *Tempora* has no singular.

---

1. 34: Isidore distinguishes between facial appearance, *vultus*, and expression, *facies*, at *Differentiarum* I. 589 [*PL* 83: 68].

1. 36: Empedocles suggested that certain particles went forth from the eyes to meet similar particles emitted by the object seen: vision resulted from their contact. Although naive, this theory made clear that vision was no mere passive reflection of external objects. See R. E. Siegel, "Theories of vision and color perception of Empedocles and Democritus," *Bulletin of the History of Medicine* 33 (1959): 145.

1. 37: *Easdem pupillas* must refer to the mires, or images, which can be seen reflected from the surface of the normal cornea—it probably does not refer to cataracts, and can hardly refer to pupillary constriction.

they are constantly in motion. They run to meet each other, as though by their assiduous activity they renewed the eyes' protection. They are fortified by a rampart of hairs, so that anything striking against [even] the opened eyes will be repelled, and when the eyes are closed in sleep, they lie hidden as though in obscurity.

40. At the margins of the lids, where they hold themselves closed, a row of hairs stands in orderly sequence, attending to the eyes' safety, lest they easily take injury from things chancing against them, and thereby be harmed. These hairs prevent contact with dust or any harsher material, and even serve to soften the air itself by diluting it, making vision bright and clear.

41. Some people think that tears, *lacrima* are named from some laceration of mind; others think that it is because the Greeks call them *DAKRUA*.

42. The coverings by which the eyes are served are called eyelids, *cilium*, because they conceal the eyes and cover them for safekeeping. The eyebrow, *supercilium*, is so named because it is placed above the eyelids, *super cilia:* these are invested with hairs that they may serve as protection for the eyes, and ward off the sweat which pours down from the forehead. The *intercilium*, however, is the hairless space between the eyebrows.

43. The cheeks, *genae*, are the parts below the eyes where the beard commences, for in Greek the beard [is] *GENEION*: hence also "cheeks," because it is here that the beard begins to grow, *gigni*.

44. The cheek bones, *mala*, are prominent parts placed under the eyes for their protection: they are called *malae* either because they protrude in roundness, which the Greeks call *MÊLA*, below the eyes, or because they are above the jawbone, *maxilla*.

45. *Maxilla* is formed as a diminutive of *mala*, just as "peg" comes from "pale" or *taxillus* from *talus*. The mandibles, *mandibulae*, are parts of the jaws, and their name comes from this. Our forefathers named the beard, *barba*, because it is proper to men, not to women.

46. The ear, *auris*, is named from the hearing of voices, whence also Vergil [*Aeneid* 4. 359]: *Vocemque his auribus ausit,* "And he heard the voice with these ears," or because the Greeks call the voice itself *AUDÊ*, from "audition"; for by changing a letter, AURES is pronounced AUDES. The voice re-echoing through their circuitous route makes the sound which the senses apprehend by hearing. The *pinnula*

is the highest part of the ear, named after "point," for the ancients called anything sharp, *pinnus*, whence we have both "'bipennate" and "pennate."

47. The nostrils, *nares*, are so named because through them either odor or spirit is not lacking to the nose, or because through odor they remind us that we may know something and understand it. For this reason and, on the other hand, the unknowing and uneducated are called "ignorant," *ignarus*. Our elders used to say that to smell was to know. Terence [*Adelphi* 397]:

> *Ac non totis sex mensibus*
> *prius olfecissent, quam ille quidquam coeperit.*

"And wouldn't they have smelled it six whole months before he started anything?"

48. The straight part of the nose which is erect and of the same length as roundness is called the column, *columna;* its end, the *pirula*, from its pear-like, *pirus*, shape; but those parts to the left and right, *pinnula*, from their resemblance to wings; the place between is the *interfinium*.

49. The mouth, *os,* is so called because through it as through a door, *ostium*, we send food inside and expel sputum; or because food enters and speech emerges there.

50. The lips are named from licking, *lambere*: the upper lip we term the *labium*, the lower, the *labrum*, because it is larger. Others say that men have *labra*, women *labia*.

51. Varro thinks that the tongue, *lingua*, was named from binding food, *ligare;* others, because it binds words together from articulated sounds, just as the tongue plays over the teeth like the plectrum of a stringed instrument, and produces the sound of the voice.

52. The Greeks call the teeth, *dentes, ODONTES,* whence the name seems to have come into Latin. The first of these are called the incisors, *praecisores*, since they first cut up everything which is taken into the mouth. Those following are the canines, *canini*, of

---

1. 42: Lewis and Short note *intercilium* as a word occurring only in lexicography, but compare with the Greek *MESOPHROUN*, the part of the skull now termed the *glabella*, and see Lactantius, *De opificio Dei* 10 [*CSEL* 27: 32–33].

1. 45: *Mandibula, -ae* and *mandibulum, -i*, seem equally correct.

1. 46: There is a more extensive discussion of the ears and their usefulness at Lactantius, *De opificio Dei* 8 [*CSEL* 27: 29–30].

1. 47: See Varro, *De lingua latina* 6. 83.

1. 48: See Lactantius, *De opificio Dei* 10 [*CSEL* 27: 33].

1. 50: Isidore differentiates between *labium* and *labrum* at *Differentiarum* I. 336 [*PL* 83: 45] along similar lines, and although neither Souter nor Lewis and Short so define *labia*, this word may have been used for the female genitalia by Isidore's time, though perhaps not in polite society. His use of *calamus* for penis at I. 1. 104 likewise draws upon a term at least colloquial.

1. 51: Ambrose, *Hexameron* 6. 66–67 [*CSEL* 32: 254–255] notes difficulty in speaking without teeth, and discusses the tongue's role in swallowing; see also Lactantius, *De opificio Dei* 11 [*CSEL* 27: 40].

1. 52: There is a similar discussion of the teeth at Lactantius, *De opificio Dei* 10 [*CSEL* 27: 35–36]. *Canini* is used chiefly in the plural, and Anibal Ruiz Moreno, *La medicina en la obra de San Isidoro* (Buenos Aires, 1950), p. 48, suggests that *columellus* is derived from *columnaris dens*.

which there are two in the right jaw and two in the left: they are called "canines" because they are considered to be similar in appearance to dogs' teeth. Dogs break bones with these, just as men do, so that the incisors hand on to them to tear what they are unable to cut themselves. The common people call these *colomelli* because of their length and roundness. The last are the molars which knead and grind and chew what has been cut by the incisors and torn by the canines: hence they are called "grinders," *molares*.

53. Gender determines the number of teeth, for they are thought to be more numerous in men, fewer in women.

54. The gums, *gingivae*, are named because they grow teeth: they were created to adorn the teeth, lest bare they might seem more of a horror than an ornament.

55. Our palate, *palatum*, is placed like the vault of heaven; "palate" is derived from "pole." The Greeks call this palate ["heaven"] *OURANOS* since in its concavity it has a resemblance to the sky.

56. The throat, *fauces*, is named from the production of sounds, or because we speak, *fari*, words through it. The windpipes, *arteriae*, are named either because air (this is the spirit) is carried through them from the lung or because they keep the vital spirit confined in the joints and narrow passages from which the voice resounds: these sounds would all be the same if the motion of the tongue did not produce a variation.

57. *Toles* are named in the Gallic tongue, and vulgarly and through diminution, they are "tonsils," *tusillas*, which often swell up in the throat. The chin is named [*mentum*, "the coping,"] because the mandibles arise or are joined together there.

58. The soft palate, *gurgulio*, derives its name from the gullet, *guttur*, whose pathway reaches to the mouth

and nostrils, [and which] has a channel through which the voice is carried to the tongue to be able to produce words. Whence we say "to be garrulous," *garrire*.

59. The esophagus, *rumen*, by which food and drink are swallowed is next to the windpipe, *gurgulio:* hence, the beasts which regurgitate their food and chew it again are said to ruminate. The epiglottis, *sublinguium,* is a lid for the windpipe and is like a small tongue which opens and closes the orifice [behind] the tongue.

60. The neck, *collum*, is so called because it is rigid and round like a column, bearing the head and holding it up like a capitol; the anterior part is called the throat, *gula;* the posterior part, the nape, *cervix.*

61. The nape, *cervix,* however is named because through that part the cerebrum is directed in a straight line to the spinal cord as through a channel for the brain. Our forefathers, however, used to say "necks" in the plural number: Hortensius better said "neck" in the singular. But "neck" in the singular number signifies the member itself, for in the plural it often indicates obstinacy. Cicero, in his oration against Verres [6. 110] says: *Praetorem tu accuses? frange cervices,* "You accuse the praetor? Curb your audacity."

62. The shoulders, *umerus*, are named as though the forequarters, *armus*, to distinguish men from mute cattle, since the former are said to have shoulders and the latter to have forequarters. For properly, "forequarters" pertain to quadrupeds. *Ola* is the posterior part of the highest part of the humerus.

63. The arms, *brachium,* are named from "strength," for in Greek, *BARUS* signifies "heavy" and "strong." There are bulges of muscles in the arms and strength is an obvious characteristic of muscles. These are bulges, *torus,* that is, muscles, and are called *torus* since the organs seem to be twisted, *tortus,* there.

64. The elbow, *cubitus,* is so named because we lean upon it when we eat. The *ulna,* according to some, is an extension of either hand, according to others, of the elbow: this seems to be the more correct interpretation, since the elbow is called *OLENE* in Greek.

1. 55. Schwarz reads *palatum nostrum, sicut caelum, est positum, et inde palatum a polo per derivationem,* and notes *nostrum* as corrupted from *sursum,* on the authority of Cicero, *De natura deorum* 2. 56. 141. In other manuscripts, Otto notes *palatum nostrum, sicut caelum, sursum est positum.* Lindsay's reading is translated.

1. 56: The trachea, *aspera arteria,* here seems to be confused with other arteries, possibly because the arterial side of the vascular tree—like the trachea—is empty after death, the veins remaining filled with blood.

1. 57: *Toles* is defined by Lewis and Short as "a goitre or wen on the neck," and is of Celtic derivation. *Tonsilla* is defined by Isidore at XIX. 2. 14 as a metal or wooden hook by which the mooring lines of ships are secured, but by Celsus (6. 10; 7. 12. 2) and Pliny (11. 37. 66) with reference to the pharyngeal tonsils. Confusion between a sebaceous cyst (a "wen") and an enlarged thyroid, or goitre, is difficult to imagine. *Toles* being a Celtic word and goitre endemic in the Celtic lands of Switzerland and bordering France, one suspects that *toles* refers to the goitre; *tonsilla* to the pharyngeal *tonsils;* and the usual *apostema* or *collectio* to the wen.

Mentum is the coping, or projecting part, of a cornice.

1. 58: *Gurgulio* can refer to the gullet or to the esophagus: here, the context suggests that it be translated as the

soft palate, including the glottis, uvula, and isthmus of the fauces.

1. 59: *Cf.* Caelius Aurelianus, *De morbis chronicis* 2. 8: *super radicem linguae, quam Graeci epiglottida vocant,* and Aurelius, *De acutis passionibus* 12 [Daremberg 707]: *broncum summae partis bronci quod latine gurgulionem dicimus.* Isidore seems to have identified this with the *rumen; cf.* Paulus 270, *rumen est pars colli qua esca devoratur, unde rumare dicitur quod nunc ruminare.*

Gurgulio thus stands for the trachea, esophagus, and oropharynx.

1. 63: The ulna is probably intended here, not the humerus.

1. 64: If *manus,* as is rarely the case in later Latin, here signifies "arm," translating the passage as "an extension of either *arm*" referring to the arm and forearm makes good sense.

65. The places under the arms are called "wings," *ala*, because the motion of the arms begins there like that of wings: some call this the *ascilla* because the arms are raised up from them, that is, they are moved; whence also a little swing, *oscillum*, is named because it is put in motion. More precisely, their edges, *ora*, are moved, for "to put in motion" is the same as "to move." Some call these "under goats," *subhircus*, since in many men, they give off an odor like goats.

66. The hand, *manus*, is so named because it is of service, *munus*, to the whole body. It gives food to the mouth, does all work and carries out all things; by it, we give and receive. By a false usage, "hand" is defined as an "employment" or "workman," whence we say "wages," *manupretium*.

67. The right hand, *dextra*, is named from giving, *dare*, because it is given in pledge of peace; it is likewise used as a witness of faith, and in greeting, and this is the case in Tully [Cicero, *Catiline* 3. 8] : *Fidem publicam iussu senatus dedi*, "By order of the senate, I have pledged the public faith," that is, the right hand. Whence also the Apostle [[Galatians 2: 9]: *Dextras dederunt mihi*, "They have given their right hands to me."]

68. The left hand, *sinixtra*, is named as though it meant "permits the right hand," *sine dextra*, or because it permits a thing to be done. The left hand is named from "permit," *sinere*.

69. The palm, *palma*, is the hand with the fingers extended, just as when the fingers are contracted, it is called the fist. "Fist," *pugnus*, is named after "pugilist," *pugillus*, as the palm is named after the spreading branches of the palm tree.

70. The digits are named either because there are ten, *decem*, of them, or because they are thought to be so properly, *decenter*, put together, constituting in themselves a perfect number and the most elegant order. The first is called the thumb, *pollex*, because it surpasses, *pollere*, the others in strength and power. The second is the *index* and greeting or demonstratory finger, because we generally greet and point out with it.

71. The third is the lewd finger, *impudicus*, since very often derision at unchaste conduct is manifested by it. The fourth is the ring finger, *anularis*, since the ring is worn on it: it is also the medicinal finger, *medicinalis*, since physicians apply salve with it. The fifth is the *auricular* finger, for we scratch our ears with it.

72. The nails, *ungula*, we name from the Greek, for they call them *ONUX*. The trunk, *truncus*, is the middle part of the body, extending from the neck to the groins. Nigidius [108] said of this: *Caput collo vehitur, truncus sustinetur coxis et genibus cruribusque*, "The head is carried by the neck, the trunk is borne up by the hips, knees and legs."

73. The anterior part of the trunk, from the neck to the stomach, is called the *thorax* by the Greeks, which we call the "ark," *arx*, because what is there is concealed, *arcanus*, that is, secret, and others are shut out. Whence both a chest, *arca*, and an altar, *ara*, are named as though they were secret things. Its soft eminences are called breasts, *mamilla*, between which is the bony part, called the breast-bone, *pectus*, with the ribs, *costa*, to the left and right.

74. Since there is a nape, *pexus*, between the prominent parts of the breasts, the breast bone, *pectus*, is so named; and a comb, *pecten*, is named because it makes the hairs smooth, *pexus*. The breasts, *mamilla*, are so called from their applelike roundness, *mala*, by diminution.

75. The nipple, *papilla*, is the prominence of the breasts, of which those sucking take hold. They are called "nipples" because infants are as though eating pap, *pappare*, when they suck milk. In the same manner the breast is all distended with abundance, but the nipple itself from which the milk is drawn is small.

76. It is called a teat, *uber*, either because filled, *uberta*, with milk or because moist, *uvida*, filled with the liquid milk as though a grape, *uva*.

77. Milk, *lac*, derives the force of its name from color, since it is a white fluid: in Greek, they say *LEUKOS* for "white." Its nature is changed out of that of blood, for after parturition, if any blood is left unused for the nourishment of the uterus, it flows in its natural channel to the breasts, and by their force becoming white, receives the qualities of milk.

---

1. 65: Essentially the same definition is repeated in another context at XX. 14. 11.
1. 66: On *manupretium*, see Varro, *De lingua latina* 5. 178.
1. 68: Lindsay's text is translated, but the manuscripts at this point are confused.
1. 71: *Insectatio* can mean "an inclination toward" and, if so, this passage would imply an inclination toward something shameful. Pressing the middle or long finger against the palm in shaking hands has certain homosexual implications, and the same finger is used as a vaguely sodomitic gesture of derision. *Cf.* Richard Burton, "Terminal Essay," *The Book of the Thousand Nights and a Night* (London, 1886, reprinted in D. W. Cory, ed., *Homosexuality: a cross-cultural approach* [New York, 1956], p. 218): "Debauchees had signals like freemasons whereby they recognized one another. The Greek Skematízein was made by closing the hand to represent the scrotum and raising the middle finger as if to feel whether a hen had eggs, *táter si les poulettes ont l'œuf:* hence the Athenians called it Catapugon or sodomite and the Roman *digitus impudicus* or *infamis*, the "medical finger" of Rabelais and the Chiromantists. Another sign was to scratch the head with the minimus—*digitulo caput scabere*."
1. 75: Isidore distinguishes still further at *Differentiarum* I. 372 [*PL* 83: 48] between male nipples (*mamillae*), female breasts (*mammae*), bovine teats (*ubera*) and the nipples (*papillae*) of a lactating breast.
1. 76: See Isidore, *Differentiarum* I. 595 [*PL* 83: 68–69].

78. The skin, *cutis,* is that which is first on the body, and is so named from its position, since it is the first to suffer in any cutting wound: a cut is called *KUTIS* in Greek. The hide, *pellis,* is the same thing, because it keeps external injuries from the body, *pellere,* warding off rains and winds and the sun's heat.

79. Directly, however, the pelt is removed, what is left is called the hide, *corium. Corium* is derived from "flesh," *caro,* which it covers, but this is proper to brute animals.

80. The pores, *porus,* of the body have a Greek name: in proper Latin, however, they are called "breathing holes," *spiramentum,* because the vivifying spirit is conducted through them outside the body.

81. *Arvina* is fat which adheres to the skin. Solid flesh, *pulpa,* is flesh without fat, so named because it palpitates, *palpitare,* for often, it springs back. Many also call this [solid flesh] the "gum," *viscus,* because it is so gluey, *glutinosus.*

82. The members are parts of the body.

83. The joints, *artus,* by which the members are bound together are named from "press together," *artare.* Sinews, *nervus,* are named by derivation from the Greek, who call them *NEURON.* Others think that they are called *nervus* in Latin because adhering one to the other they provide for the articulation of joints. It is most certain that sinews make up the greatest part of men's strength, for the more solid they are, the more apt they are to increase bodily strength.

84. The joints, *artus,* are so named because they move whilst bound together, that is, while held tightly together by sinews: the diminutive of this is "articulation," *articulus.* We say "joints" when referring to the greater members, such as arms, but "articulations" when speaking of lesser members, such as fingers.

85. The heads of the bones are called a "joint," *conpago,* because pressed, *conpacta,* to each other by the sinews, they stick together as though by some glue.

86. The bones, *os,* form the foundations of the body; posture and all strength is based on them. The bones are named from "burnt," *ustus,* since the ancients burned them or, as others think, from the mouth, *os,* since they can be seen there, for they are hidden and covered over by viscera or skin everywhere else.

87. The marrow, *medulla,* is so named because it moistens the bones, irrigating and strengthening them. The vertebrae, *vertibulum,* are the end parts of the bones, pressed together by large nodes and named because they are rotated, *vertere,* for the motion of the members.

88. Cartilages are soft bones without marrow: the ear, the nasal septum and the ends of the ribs have this kind [of bone], or which forms a covering for moving bones. They are called *cartilago* since a light rubbing is painless when they are bent.

89. Some think that the ribs, *costa,* are named because they guard the internal parts of the body and, surrounded by them, the whole soft part of the belly is kept safe.

90. The side, *latus,* is so named because it is hidden when we lie down, for it is the left side of the body. The right side is more nimble in movement; the left is stronger and better adapted for bearing a burden. The left is also named because it is more apt for lifting, *levare,* and carrying anything. For it is the left side which bears the shield, sword, quiver, and other burdens, leaving the right hand unimpeded for action.

91. The back, *dorsum,* extends from the neck to the loins, *renes:* it is called the back because it is the harder, *durior,* surface of the body, much like a stone, and is strong for carrying and suffering patiently.

92. The back sides, *terga,* are so named because we lie on them supine on the earth, *terra,* which man alone can do: the brute animals lie either on their bellies or on their sides. For this reason, *tergum* is wrongly used when speaking of animals.

93. The *scapula* [. . .] The *interscapilium* is the space between the scapulae, whence its name.

94. The "spades," *palae,* are prominent parts of the back, right and left, so named because in wrestling, which the Greeks call *PALE,* we press them down.

95. The spine, *spina,* is the name given to the joints of the back, so named because it has sharp

---

1. 78: This passage has caused much editorial concern with the Greek *KUTOS,* "skin," equivalent to the Latin *cutis:* Isidore incorrectly defines *KUTIS* as "cut."

1. 79: This seems to refer to the panniculus carnosus of the lower animals, surviving in man only as the rudimentary platysma muscle: Isidore's comparative anatomy is correct. *Corium* is defined at Servius Daniel *Aeneid* 1. 211.

1. 80: In later Latin generally, *spiramentum* referred to a human breath; here it is "breathing pore," as in classical Latin.

1. 81: See Servius *Aeneid* 7. 627.

1. 83: Until much later than Isidore's time, the difference between nerves and tendons was rarely appreciated, although functional differences were appreciated in concrete cases, and both were termed *nervi.* This confusion will be appreciated by anyone who has attempted to repair a laceration of the wrist.

1. 85: See Lactantius, *De opificio Dei* 5 [CSEL 27: 20].

1. 86: *Os,* "bone," but *ōs,* "mouth"; for an account of the skeleton as the body's foundation, see Lactantius, *De opificio Dei* 7 [CSEL 27: 24].

1. 87: This passage may refer to the union between the epiphysis and the diaphysis.

1. 88: There is a long discussion of the various kinds of joints at Lactantius, *De opificio Dei* 5 [CSEL 27: 20–21].

1. 90: The phrase *quia jacentibus nobis latet* admits of two interpretations: "since it is hidden when we lie down" or "since it protects us from missiles."

1. 91: *Renes* is used in the plural and *ren* is a synthetic form.

1. 92: See *Differentiarum* I. 562 [PL 83: 66].

1. 95: See Lactantius, *De opificio Dei* 5 [CSEL 27: 19].

little rays; its joints are called "spondyles," *spondilium,* because of the part of the brain which is carried through them by a long passageway to other parts of the body.

96. The sacral spine, *sacra spina,* is the termination of the continuous part of the spine, and the Greeks call this bone *HIERON OSTOUN;* because it is the first part which develops in an infant after conception, likewise since it is the first part of the sacrificial animal offered by the pagans to their gods, whence also it is called the "sacred bone."

97. Varro says that the kidneys, *renes,* are so named because the stream, *rivus,* of semen, *obscenus humor,* arises therefrom. The veins and spinal cord, *medulla,* sweat out a thin fluid into the kidneys and this fluid, redissolved by venereal heat, runs down from the kidneys.

98. The loins, *lumbus,* are named from the lewdness of lust, *libido,* since the seat of bodily pleasure is located there in men, just as it is in the umbilicus in women. Thus it is said to Job [38: 3] at the beginning of the speech: *Accinge sicut vir lumbos tuos,* "Gird up your loins like a man," as though preparation to resist were located in the same places where the usual source of lust's domination resides.

99. The *umbilicus* is the central part of the body, named because it is the prominent part of the flanks, *umbus iliorum;* and for the same reason, the place in the middle of a shield by which it hangs is called the *umbo.* The infant hangs from its umbilicus in the womb, and is also nourished through it.

100. The groin, *ilium,* has a Greek name because we cover ourselves up at that place, for in Greek, †*ilios*† is said for "wrap around."

101. The buttocks, *clunes,* are so named because they are near the great gut, *colum,* which is the "straight gut," *longao;* the *nates* because when we sit, we bear down on them, *inniteri.* For this reason, flesh is concentrated there, lest the bones suffer pain from the weight of the body.

---

1. 96: For discussions of the *HIERON OSTOUN* (or *OSTEON*), see Caelius Aurelianus, *De morbis chronicis* 4. 3 and Suetonius, "Deperditorum librorum reliquiae" (Roth 302).

1. 97: See Varro, *De lingua latina* 5. 126 and Lactantius, *De opificio Dei* 14 [*CSEL* 27: 48–49], and see notes on XI. 1. 103–104 below. *Medulla* here refers to the *medulla spinalis,* or spinal cord.

1. 99: There is a full discussion of omphalology at Varro, *De lingua latina* 7. 17.

1. 100: Lindsay has placed †*ilios*† between daggers as a mark of textual corruption, probably rightly. The manuscripts variously read *ilios* or *ileos;* Arevalo, reprinted by Migne, suggests *EILUEIN,* and others have offered *HEILISSEIN,* without manuscript authority. Perhaps *ileos* is correct, and Isidore confuses *ilium* with the disease *ileos,* colic: see IV. 6. 14, and the note thereon.

1. 101: *Clunes* is usually used in the plural; singular, *clunis. Cf.* Lactantius, *De opificio Dei* 13 [*CSEL* 27: 47]: *Conglobata in nates caro, quam sedendi officio apta!* *Longao* is the "straight gut," the *intestinum rectum.*

102. The *genitalia* are parts of the body, as the name itself shows, which have taken a name from the generation of offspring, procreated and given birth by these parts. They are also called *pudenda* from "modesty," *verecundia,* or because of the hair which appears on the body at the age of puberty: we cover these parts with clothing for the same reason. Those some [parts] are also called the "unchaste parts" since they lack the same decent appearance as the members placed before the eyes.

103. The penis, *veretrum,* is so named because it is "proper to a man," *viri est tantum,* or because semen, *virus,* is emitted from it; for *virus,* properly speaking, is the fluid which comes from the male organs of generation.

104. The testis, *testiculus,* is named by diminution from "witness," *testis,* and their number commences at two. These supply semen which comes from the spinal cord, kidneys, and loins to the penis, *calamus,* for the purpose of procreation. The scrotum, *fiscus,* is the skin within which the testes are located.

105. The posterior parts are indeed so named because they are behind, turned away from the face, lest we be offended by the sight as we empty our bowels. The opening, *meatus,* is so called because the feces go through it, *meare,* that is, they are forced through it.

106. The thighs, *femur,* are so named because by these parts, the male gender is distinguished from the female: they extend from the groins to the knees. *Femina* is a derivation, referring to the parts of the thighs by which we hold on to a horse's back when riding. Whence in olden times, fighters were said to have lost their horses from between their thighs.

107. The hips, *coxa,* are similar to *axes* which have been joined together, for the thighs are moved by them. Their joints are called "concave" because the heads of the thigh bones are turned in them. The hollow of the knee, *suffrago,* is named because bent, i.e., broken, *subitus frangere,* underneath and not bent upward as the arms.

108. The knees, *genu,* are the junctures of the thighs and the legs, and they are named "knees" because while in the womb they are opposite the cheeks, *gena,* where they are close together and, cognate with the eyes, indices of tears and of mercy. For the knees are named after the cheeks.

109. Finally, man is shaped and formed folded so that his knees are erect by which his eyes are formed

---

1. 103: *Virus* in classical Latin generally is any slimy fluid, and need not pertain only to semen.

1. 104: The *testes* witness to manliness, since a castrated man had certain civil disabilities at Roman law.

1. 105: *Meatus* refers to any natural opening in the human body.

1. 106: *Femina* here is the nominative plural of *femen, -inis;* compare with the English "his horse shot from under him."

so that they are round and hidden. Ennius [*Inc.* 14]: *Atque genua conprimit arta gena,* "And presses together the cheek close to bent knees." Hence it is that when men cast themselves upon their knees, they begin straightway to weep. For nature wants them to recall their mothers' wombs, where they sat as though in utter darkness before they came into the light of day.

110. The legs, *crus,* are named because we walk and run, *currere,* on them: they extend downward from the knees to the ankles. The tibias, *tibia,* are named as though "flutes," *tuba*—they are similar in length and in appearance.

111. The ankle, *talus,* is named from the ankle bone, *tolus,* in that the ankle bone is a round prominence, whence also the top point in a circular shrine is called the *tolus.* But the ankle is behind the shin, under the ankle bone of the heel.

112. The feet, *pes,* are given a name from Greek etymology, for the Greeks call them *POUS,* [things] which walk with alternate steps upon the firm earth.

113. The sole, *planta,* is named from "flatness," *planities,* since they are not rounded as in quadrupeds, lest men be unable to stand on two feet, but they are formed long and flat to make the body stable. However, there are anterior parts of the sole which are also made up of many bones.

114. The heel, *calcis,* is the proximal part of the sole: the name is from the thick skin, *callus,* with which we tread, *calcare,* the earth, hence also "heel," *calcaneus.*

115. The sole, *solum,* is the under side of the foot, named because with it we impress our footprints on the ground. Everything, however, which holds anything else up is also called *solum,* as though it were solid: whence the earth also is termed *solum,* since it sustains everything, and the sole of the foot, because it carries the whole weight of the body.

116. We say *viscera* not only with reference to the intestines, but to whatever is under the skin, from the "gum," *viscus,* which is between skin and flesh. Likewise, the viscera are "vitals," *vitalia,* that is, placed all around the heart, as though "vigor of the heart," *viscora,* since life, that is, the soul, is centered there.

117. Similarly, the heads of the sinews, made of blood and nerves plaited together, are called *viscera.* Again, [muscles] are termed "lizards," *lacertus,* or "mice," *mus,* because these animals have the equivalent of a heart all throughout their several members so that the heart is the center of the whole body, and they are called by the name of similar animals which hide themselves under the earth. Hence, muscles, *musculus,* are named from a similarity to sea-mice, *mus,* and are likewise called *torus,* because the organs seem twisted, *tortus,* in these places.

118. Heart, *cor,* is derived from the Greek name, because they say *KARDIA,* or from "care," *cura,* for therein resides all solicitude and concern for knowledge. It is therefore near the lung so that when it flames up with wrath, it may be tempered by the lung's humor. This has two channels, *arteria,* of which the left has more blood, the right, more vital spirit. Whence also we feel the pulse in the right arm.

119. The *praecordia* are the places near the heart by which sensation is perceived, and are called the *praecordia* because there is located the source, *principium,* of the heart and of cogitation.

120. The pulse, *pulsus,* is named because it palpitates: from its indications we learn concerning sickness or health. Its motion is duplex, either simple or composite. The simple, which is marked by one pace; the composite, which is irregular and unequal because of many motions. This motion has definite intervals: striking dactylically so long as there is no disorder, but whenever it is more rapid, as *DORKADAZONTES,* or more feeble, as *MURMIZONTES,* it is a mortal sign.

121. Veins, *vena,* are named because they are channels, *via,* of flowing blood, and are divided into streams throughout the entire body, by which all the members are irrigated.

122. Blood, *sanguis,* gets its name from the Greek etymology, since it is so active, sustaining and giving life. It is, however, blood while in the body, but once spilled out it is called "gore," *cruor.* For it is gore because it gushes down in a stream, or because it sinks to the ground in a flux. Others think that gore refers to corrupt blood which is discharged; still others say that blood is so named because it is sweet, *suavis.*

123. Except in youth, the blood is not unexhausted, *integer,* for physicians say that the blood supply is diminished with age, whence also tremor occurs in the elderly; but properly, blood is controlled by the soul, for which reason women customarily scratch their cheeks in grief, whence also purple clothing and purple flowers are furnished the dead.

---

1. 111: This description fits the os calcaneus, or astralgus.

1. 113: *Sura* may refer to the calf of the leg, or to the fibula; see also *Differentiarum* I. 546 [*PL* 83: 65].

1. 115: See Servius *Aeneid* 7. 111.

1. 116: *Cf.* Servius *Aeneid* 1. 215: *viscera non tantum intestina dicimus, sed quicquid sub corio est.*

1. 117: The *mus* from which *musculus,* "muscle," is derived was an eel of some kind, not the familiar rodent, hence the use of *lacertus,* "lizard," for muscle.

1. 120: See Appendix A, "A Note on the Pulse."

1. 121: See Lactantius, *De opificio Dei* 7 [*CSEL* 27: 24–25].

1. 122: Henry Nettleship, *Lectures and essays* (Oxford, 1885), pp. 358–359, quotes Placidus, and comments: "This gloss looks like a corrupt abbreviation of a note in which tabus, cruor, and sanguis were distinguished." Isidore repeats the distinction at *Differentiarum* I. 529 [*PL* 83: 63].

1. 123: See Servius *Aeneid* 9. 255; on the use of purple for mourning, see Servius Daniel *Aeneid* 3. 67.

124. The lung, *pulmo*, derives a name from the Greek, for the Greeks call the lung *PLEUMON*, since it is a fan for the heart, in which the *PNEUMA*, that is, the [vital] spirit, is centered, by which they are both set in motion and moved; whence also the lungs are named. For in Greek, the [vital] spirit is called *PNEUMA*, which by blowing up and stirring, sends out and takes in the air by which the lungs are moved and palpitate, and opening themselves to catch a breath, contracting to expel it. It is an organ of the body.

125. The liver, *iecur*, is so named because the fire, *ignis*, which flies up to the brain has a seat there. It diffuses from there to the eyes, the other senses and members; and by its own heat changes the juice, *sucus*, which it draws to itself from food into blood, which it provides for the nourishment and sustenance of each member. Pleasure and sensual desire have their seats in the liver, according to those who dispute concerning scientific matters.

126. The ends of the liver are pointed, as [also] the ends of endive leaves, or like tongues sticking out. They are called "entrails," *fibra*, because among the pagans, in rites at the altars of Phoebus, responses were given by soothsayers, *ferebantur ab ariolis*, who received their answers when the livers were sacrificed and burned.

127. The spleen, *splen*, is named since it serves as a supplement in the part opposite the liver, lest the space be empty. Some also think that it was made as a source for laughter, for we laugh with the spleen, are angry with the bile, understand with the heart and love with the liver. The whole animal is made up of these four fixed elements.

128. Gall, *fel*, is so named since there is a little bag, *folliculum*, which contains the humor called bile, *bilis*. The mouth, *stomachus*, is called *os* in Greek since it is

the door to the belly, and it takes the food and passes it into the intestine.

129. The intestines, *intestinum*, are so named because located in the inner parts of the body, arranged in long circular entwinings, so that the food swallowed can gradually be digested, and not impeded by food swallowed later.

130. The *omentum*, which the Greeks call *EPIPLOON*, is a membrane containing the greater part of the intestines. The diaphragm, *disseptum intestinum*, separates the stomach and other intestines from the lungs [and] from the heart.

131. The blind intestine, *caecum*, which the Greeks call *TUPHLON ENTERON*, is named because it is without aperture or egress. The small intestine, *jejuna*, is the narrowest of the intestines, whence also we say "fast day," *jejunium*.

132. The belly, *venter*, bowel, *alvus*, and womb, *uterus*, differ one from another: the belly is that which digests the food which has been eaten, it can be seen from without and extends from the breast to the groin and is called the belly since it transmits life's nourishment, *vitae alimenta*, throughout the whole body.

133. The bowel is that which receives food, and which is customarily purged. Sallust [*Historiae* I, frag. 52]: *Simulans sibi alvum purgari*, "Pretending that he purged his bowel." It is also called the bowel because it is cleansed, that is, purged, for from it flows the filth of the feces.

134. Only women have a womb, which resembles the stalk of a plant, *cauliculum*, and within which they conceive. Nevertheless, some authors—not just poets, but others as well—would like a "womb" for both sexes, and many write "belly" for this organ.

135. It is called the *uterus* because it is double and divides itself into two parts which spread in differing directions opposite each other and bend around very much like a ram's horn, or because inside it is filled

---

1. 124: For accounts of the cooling effect of the lungs on the heart's passions, see Augustine, *De anima* 2. 4 [*PL* 44: 573]; Lactantius, *De opificio Dei* 11 [*CSEL* 27: 39]; and Ambrose, *Hexameron* 6. 70 [*CSEL* 32: 257–258]. William Harvey, *De motu cordis* 36, has similar views.

1. 125: The liver is the warmest organ of the body at rest, and is exceeded in temperature only by actively contracting skeletal muscle. Fletcher, *op. cit.*, p. 80, notes: "In a passage in the *Differ.* II. 16, 17, fire has its seat in the liver, thence it flies to the head as to the heavens of the body. From this fire come the rays which flash from the eyes, and from the middle of this fire, narrow passages lead not only to the eyes but also to the other senses." On the hepatic localization of libido and of digestion, see also Servius *Aeneid* 6. 596, and Lactantius, *De opificio Dei* 14 [*CSEL* 27: 49].

1. 126: See Servius Daniel *Georgics* 1. 120; Servius *Georgics* 1. 120; and Servius *Aeneid* 10. 176.

1. 127: The function of the spleen was poorly understood in ancient times, but was assigned a role in the production of black bile. See Ambrose, *Hexameron* 6. 71 [*CSEL* 32: 258].

1. 128: Lindsay queries *os*, mouth, or *OISOPHAGOS*, esophagus: either would fit the description.

1. 129: See Lactantius, *De opificio Dei* 11 [*CSEL* 27: 41–42].

1. 130: *Cf.* Pseudo-Soranus, *Quaestiones medicinales* 243 [Rose 272]: *peritonium id est omentum quo intestina circumdata sunt*, which suggests that the nouns *omentum* and *peritoneum* were used for the same object. Ruiz Moreno, *op. cit.*, p. 63, identifies *omentum* here with the mesentery, probably incorrectly. Dressel, pp. 265–266, refers this passage to an anonymous scholiast on Lucan 1. 625, and derives XI. 1. 130–134 from the same source.

1. 131: See Varro, *De lingua latina* 5. 111.

1. 132: Isidore again distinguishes between *alvus*, *venter*, and *uterus* at *Differentiarum* I. 38 [*PL* 83: 14–15].

1. 134: Could Isidore have Ambrose in mind? *Cf. Hexameron* 6. 71 [*CSEL* 32: 258]: *conficitur primum esca in utero superiore, deinde in jecore coquitur*.

1. 135: This probably refers to a bicornuate uterus, not an uncommon developmental anomaly in human beings and the rule in lower animals; a "ram's horn" is an appropriate description of a uterus with attached adnexa involved by chronic gonorrheal salpingitis, a disease not rare in women whose bodies come to public dissection.

with the fetus. Hence also [it is called] the "pouch," *uter,* because it has something inside, members and viscera.

136. The "paunch," *aqualiculus,* properly pertains to the pig, hence its transposition to "belly," *venter.* It is called the *matrix* since the fetus arises therein: it carefully cherishes the semen which it has received, and fashions what it has warmed into a body, drawing this embodied mass out into members.

137. The *vulva* is named by analogy to a folding door, *valva,* that is, the door of the belly, because it receives the semen, or because the fetus proceeds from it. The bladder, *vesica,* is named as though a "water vessel," *vas aqua,* thus, it is filled by urine collected from the kidneys, and is distended by fluid. It does not have this function in birds.

138. Urine, *urina,* is named either because it burns, *urere,* or because it is collected from the kidneys. Its indication is a prognosis of both future health and disease. The urine is vulgarly called *lotium* because by its use clothing may be made *lotum,* that is, clean.

139. Seed, *semen,* is that which once sown, is taken up either by the earth or by the womb for the generation of fruit or fetus. It is a liquid made through a decoction of food and of the body and spread through the veins and spinal cord whence, sweated out in the manner of bilge-water, it condenses in the kidneys. Ejaculated during coitus and taken up in the woman's womb, it is shaped in the body of a certain visceral heat and the humidity of the menstrual blood.

140. The menstrual flow is a woman's superfluous blood: it is termed "menstrual," *menstrua,* because of the phase of the light of the moon by which this flow comes about. The moon is called *MĒNĒ* in Greek. These are also called the "womanlies," *muliebria,* for woman is the only menstrual animal.

141. On contact with this gore, crops do not germinate, wine goes sour, grasses die, trees lose their fruit, iron is corrupted by rust, copper is blackened. Should dogs eat any of it, they go mad. Even bituminous glue, which is dissolved neither by iron nor by [strong] waters, polluted by this gore, falls apart by itself.

142. After many menstrual days, however, the semen is no longer germinable because there is no menstrual blood by which the ejaculate can be irrigated. Thin semen does not adhere to the female parts; lacking this power to adhere, it is lost. Likewise, thick semen also lacks the power of growth, being unable to mix with the female blood because of its own excessive thickness. This is why men or women become sterile: from excessive thickness of semen or blood, or from excessive thinness.

143. They say that the human heart is the first part of the body to be formed, because in it is all life and wisdom; then, by the fortieth day, the whole task is made up. This has been learned, they say, from abortions. Others say that the fetus begins to develop at the head, whence also we see in eggs that the eyes are the first parts to be formed in the fetus of birds.

144. The fetus, *foetus,* is named since it is still nourished, *fovere,* in the womb; its afterbirth, *secundae,* is called the "sac," *folliculus,* which is born at the same time as the infant and which encloses him: it is so called because when he comes forth, it also follows.

145. They say that children resemble their fathers if the paternal seed be stronger; the mother if the maternal seed be the stronger. This is the reason faces are formed to resemble others; those with the likeness of both parents were conceived from an equal admixture of paternal and maternal semen. Those resembling their grandparents and great-grandparents do so since, just as there are many seeds hidden in the soil, seeds also lie hidden in us which will give back the figures of our ancestors. Girls are born from the paternal semen and boys from the maternal, because every birth consists of two seeds. When its greater part prevails, it produces a similarity of sex.

146. In our body, certain things are made only for utility, such as the viscera; certain for both utility and beauty, as the senses on the face or the hands and feet on the body, the usefulness of these members is great, and their appearance is most becoming.

147. Certain things are for appearance's sake only, as breasts in men, and the umbilicus in either sex. Some are for the purpose of differentiation, as the genitalia, the long beard, and the wide chest in men; in women, a gentle face and a narrow chest, but for

Hippocrates, *Aphorisms* 5. 62–63. Owsei Temkin, *Soranus' Gynecology* (Baltimore, 1956) reviews the subject thoroughly.

1. 143: Alcmaeon of Croton taught that the fetal head was first formed in the uterus so that it might partake of nourishment, but the early formation of the fetal heart was common knowledge from the time of the Corpus Hippocraticum downward. See also, Lactantius, *De opificio Dei* 12 [*CSEL 27*: 44] for a short account of patristic views on embryology. Isidore here contradicts XI. 1. 96.

1. 145: See Lucretius, *De rerum natura* 4. 1209–1232, which very strongly suggests this passage. There is a long review of conception in Tertullian, *De anima* 27 [Waszink 38–39] and see Lactantius, *De opificio Dei* 12 [*CSEL 27*: 44–45] for an account of the inheritance of physical characteristics. Belief in a female semen, necessary for fertilization, persisted until the discovery of the ovum.

---

1. 137: Isidore's comment that the avian air-bladder does not have the same function as the human urinary bladder is correct; see also Lactantius, *De opificio Dei* 11 [*CSEL 27*: 42–43].

1. 138: Uroscopy was an important diagnostic tool, although in ancient times more used in prognosis than in what would now be considered diagnosis.

1. 139: See Lactantius, *De opificio Dei* 12 [*CSEL 27*: 43].

1. 141: Pliny, *Historia naturalis* 7. 15 reports the same views on menstrual blood. "Waters" refers to various acids and solvents.

1. 142: See Lucretius, *De rerum natura* 6. 1239–1247, for a review on ancient theories on sterility, and see also

conceiving and carrying young, their loins and sides are wider. What pertains to man and to the parts of his body has, in part, been said, and I shall now discuss the ages of his life.

2. THE AGES OF MAN

1. The stages of life are six: infancy, childhood, adolescence, youth, maturity, and old age.

2. The first age is infancy, *infantia*, extending from the child's birth into the light of day until the age of seven years.

3. The second age is childhood, *pueritia*, that is, pure and not yet old enough to reproduce, and lasts until the fourteenth year.

4. The third is adolescence, *adolescentia*, an age mature enough for reproduction, lasting until the twenty-eighth year.

5. The fourth, youth, *juventus*, is the strongest of all the ages, and ends with the fiftieth year.

6. The fifth age is that of riper years, that is to say, of mature judgment, *gravitas*, and is the gradual decline from youth into old age: the individual is no longer young, but he is not yet an old man. It is that period of life's maturity which the Greeks call *PRES-BUTĒS*, for an old man among the Greeks is not called an "elder," *presbyter*, but *GERŌN*. This age commences with the fiftieth year and ends with the seventieth.

7. Old age, *senectus*, is the sixth stage and is bounded by no definite span of years, but whatever of life remains after those earlier five stages is marked up to old age.

8. Senility, *senium*, is the final part of old age, so named because it is the terminus of the sixth age, *sextae aetas*. The philosophers have distributed human life among these six periods, within which limits it is changed and goes on and finally comes to its end, which is death. Let us continue briefly through the above-mentioned stages of life, pointing out their etymologies in so far as man is concerned.

9. A human being in the first stage is called an "infant," *infans*, because the infant at this stage is still unable to speak, that is, he is unable to talk. His teeth are not yet properly arranged and, as a result, his clarity of speech is limited.

10. Boy, *puer*, is named from "purity," *puritas*, because the boy is pure, not yet even having down on his rosy cheeks. These are the *ephebi*, named after Phoebus, who, not yet [grown] men are still gentle youths.

11. The word "boy" is used in three ways: referring to birth, as in Isaiah [9. 6]: *Puer natus est nobis*, "A son is born to us"; to indicate age, as "a boy eight years old," or "a ten yearling"—this is the origin of that phrase, *Iam puerile jugum tenera cervice gerebat*, "he was already bearing the boyish yoke on tender neck"; and to refer to compliance and purity of faith, as the Lord said to the Prophet [Jeremiah 1: 7]: *Puer meus es tu, noli timere*, "You are my son: do not be afraid," although Jeremiah had long since passed the years of his boyhood.

12. A girl, *puella*, is a little one, *parvula*, as though "pure," *pulla*. That is why we speak of them as "pupils," not from their pupillary status, but in view of their childish age. "Pupils," *pupillus*, however are so named, that is, "destitute of parents," as though [those] of the eyes. Properly speaking, those whose fathers died before they received their names from them are called "pupils." Others call those bereft of parents, *orbus*, "orphans," *orphanus*, which means the same as "pupil": the former is the Greek name, the latter Latin, as also in the Psalm, where we read [10: 14]: *Pupillo tu eris adjutor*, "You will be a helper of the orphaned"; the Greek has *ORPHANOS*.

13. The pubescent, *puberis*, is named from the *pubes*, that is, from the body's parts of generation, because this place then first shows the downy hairs of puberty. There are some who calculate puberty from age, reckoning that individual to be pubescent who has completed fourteen years, even though he may reach puberty very late; but most certainly anyone who shows its signs on his body and can beget children has reached puberty.

14. Lying-in women, *puerpera*, are those who bear children during their youthful years, whence Horace

2. 1: For discussions of the various ages of human life and their humoral relations, see Pseudo-Soranus, *Quaestiones medicinales* 65 [Rose 256]; Galen, *Definitiones medicae* 104 [Kühn 19: 373–374]; and Servius *Aeneid* 5. 295.

2. 6: At *Differentiarum* II. 75 [PL 83: 81], Isidore considers youth the age of greatest intellectual and physical maturity, ending at forty-nine in men and with the menopause in women.

2. 7: See *Differentiarum* I. 531 [PL 83: 63–64].

2. 9: See Varro, *De lingua latina* 6. 52.

2. 10: Arevalo cites a fragment of Varro preserved by Censorinus: *pueri, quod sint puri, id est, impuberes*, an unhappy commentary on humanity.

2. 11: See *Differentiarum* I. 460 [PL 83: 57].

2. 12: *Pupilli*, in classical times, were children whose fathers died before formally acknowledging paternity, usually by picking the child up in the presence of witnesses and placing him on his lap.

2. 13: Tertullian, *De anima* 38. 1 [Waszink 54–55] argues for a spiritual puberty at fourteen, consistent with the usual age for Christian confirmation and comparable rites in other religions. At Roman law, certain privileges were assumed at puberty, which was determined by physical changes or by the fourteenth birthday, whichever came first.

2. 14: See also *Differentiarum* I. 448 [PL 83: 55] where Isidore repeats the definition of *puerpera*, and implies that the word refers to a woman who has just been delivered of her [especially first] child, or to a girl who had borne a child when younger than usual.

[*Odes* 4. 5. 23]: *Laudatur primo prole puerpera* [*nato*], "The young mother is praised for her first male issue," and those are also called *puerpera* who are either heavy with their first child, or whose first-born are sons.

15. An adolescent, *adolescens,* is so named because he is sufficiently grown up to beget, or because he is maturing and increasing in size.

16. A young man, *juvenis,* is named because at that age he begins to be able to help, *juvare,* as a young bullock, *juvencus,* is named when he withdraws from among the calves. A young man is in that very age when energy increases, and he is already prepared to help, since it is a man's duty to devote himself to usefulness. Just as the thirtieth year is that of perfected age in man, so also the third is the strongest year in cattle and beasts of burden.

17. A man, *vir,* is named because there is greater force, *vis,* in him than in women, whence also "strength," *virtus,* takes its name, or because he rules over woman by force.

18. Woman, *mulier,* is named from "softness," *mollities,* as though "softer," *mollier,* with a letter changed and one taken away were "woman," *mulier.*

19. Both differ in bodily strength and weakness, the man's strength being greater, the woman's less, so that she may be subject to the man lest, women having repelled a man, lust may not drive him to strive after another woman, or to fall upon his own sex.

20. Woman is named according to her feminine sex, not according to a corruption of integrity, and this is clear from the language of Sacred Scripture, since Eve was made directly from her husband's side, and was forthwith named "woman," as Scripture says, without yet having been touched by a man [Genesis 2: 23]: *Et formavit eam in mulierem,* "And he formed her into a woman."

21. A virgin, *virgo,* is named from the green freshness, *viridior,* of her age, as is also a sapling, *virga,* or a calf, *vitula.* Others hold that it is from "incorruption," as a virago, since she does not yet know womanly passion.

22. A *virago* is so named because she does manly things, *virum agere,* that is, she does a man's work, and her strength is masculine. The ancients thus named strong women. But a virgin is not properly called a *virago* if she does not exercise the office of a

man, although if a woman really does a man's work, as an Amazon, she is rightly called a *virago.*

23. She whom we now call "woman," *femina,* was called *vira* by the ancients, as *serva* is derived from *servus,* or handmaiden, *famula,* from servant, *famulus,* so also *vira* from *vir.* Some think that the name "virgin," *virgo,* has the same origin.

24. The word *femina* is derived from those parts of the thighs by which this sex is distinguished from men. Others think that *femina* is derived by a Greek etymology from "fiery force," because she lusts so strongly, for the female is much more sensual than the male, among women just as among animals. Hence, love beyond measure among the ancients was called "womanly love," *femineus amor.*

25. The elder, *senior,* is still more vigorous. In the sixth book, Ovid writes [*Metamorphoses* 12. 464]:

Senior,
Inter juvenemque senemque.

"The elder, between youth and old age"; and *Terence* [*Hecyra,* II Prologue line 3]: *Quo jure sum us*[*us*] *adulescentior,* "By the same law which I used when I was younger."

26. [More adolescent] not as meaning "more than an adolescent," but less [younger]; as an elder is less of an old man since, in this case, the comparative form indicates less than the positive form, therefore, not extremely old, just as in the case of a younger man among men, or as a poor man stands between a wealthy man and a pauper.

27. The aged, *senis,* are thought by some to have been named from a diminution of sense, because through advanced age, men act foolishly. For physicians say that fools are men of colder blood, wise men of hot: hence, old men, in whom the blood has become cold, and children, in whom it has not yet become warm, have less wisdom. It is in this that old age and infancy are alike: old men lose their wits from advanced age, children do not know what they are about because of playfulness and immaturity.

28. "Old man," *senex,* however, is only of the masculine gender, just as "old wife," *anus,* is feminine, for only a woman is called an "old wife." *Anus* is named from "many years old," *annosa,* as though she were heavy with years. If the name were common in gender, why would Terence say [*Eunuchus* 357]: *senem mulierem,* "old woman"? Hence also, a "little old woman," *vetula,* because she is aged, *vetustus.* Just as extreme old age is named from the word for

---

2. 17: See Cicero, *Tusculanarum disputationum* 2. 18. 43 and Lactantius, *De opificio Dei* 12 [*CSEL* 27: 46].

2. 18: Lactantius, *De opificio Dei* 12 [*CSEL* 27: 46] cites Varro as an authority for an identical derivation of the word *mulier* from *mollier.*

2. 20: Isidore rejects Aristotle's view that it is from defect or incapacity that the female is female; see Aristotle, *De generatione animalium* 1. 20 [728a17 ff.].

2. 21: See Servius *Eclogues* 3. 30 and *Differentiarum* I. 590 [*PL* 83: 68].

2. 22: See Servius *Aeneid* 12. 468 and Genesis 2: 23.

2. 24: Isidore is more concise at *Differentiarum* I. 261 [*PL* 83: 37]: *feminam de homine, femina femora sunt.*

2. 25: Otto suggests that this citation is from a gloss on Ovid, *Metamorphoses* 12. 464, since the modern texts do not include the word *senior.*

2. 26: A similar discussion, attributed to Varro, is found at Servius *Aeneid* 5. 409.

2. 27: See Servius *Aeneid* 2. 639.

"old man," *senex,* so also "old wifehood," *anilitas,* is named from "old woman."

29. Hoariness, *canities,* is named from "glossy whiteness," *candor,* as though it were "shining," *candities.* Hence the phrase, *florida juventus, lactea canities,* "blooming youth, milky old age," as though it were to say "white."

30. Old age, moreover, brings with it much both good and bad. Good, since it frees us from the most unbridled masters, imposes moderation upon pleasures, checks the onslaught of lust, increases wisdom and imparts riper counsel. Bad also, because the greatest curse of the elderly is weakness and tedium, for [Vergil, *Georgics* 3. 67]: *subeunt morbi tristisque senectus,* "Disease and sad old age draw nigh." There are two things by which the bodily faculties are depleted, old age and illness.

31. Death, *mors,* is so named because it is bitter, *amarus,* or from Mars, who is the agent of deaths [or death is named from that bite, *morsus,* of the first man, because biting the fruit of the forbidden tree, he became subject to death].

32. There are three kinds of death: premature, *acerbus;* untimely, *inmaturus;* natural. Premature of infants, untimely of young men, earned—that is, natural—of old men.

33. It is uncertain according to which part of speech the word "dead," *mortuus,* should be inflected for, as Caesar said, if it is from *morior,* in the participle of the past tense, it ought to end in TUS, with only one U, not two, for when the letter U is doubled, it is nominative and not participial, as in *fatuus, arduus.* Consequently, it happens suitably that inasmuch as it cannot be explained what it means in reality to die, it cannot be said how the word ought to be inflected in speaking.

34. Every dead man is either a corpse, *funus,* or a *cadaver:* the body is a corpse if it be buried, and a funeral is named from the burning fumes of wax-impregnated reeds which formerly were carried before the bier.

35. Should the body be unburied, it is a *cadaver,* for a *cadaver* is named from "falling down," *cadere,* because it is no longer able to stand. While the body is carried, we say "exsequial," *exsequialis,* when consumed by fire, "reliquial," *reliquialis,* and when buried, "sepulchral," *sepultus.* "Body," *corpus,* is customarily

said, as that [phrase] [Vergil, *Georgics* 4. 255]: *tum corpora luce carentum,* "the bodies of those lacking light."

36. One is called "defunct," *defunctus,* because he has finished the duties of life, for we use the expression "he retired from his post," *functus officio,* of people who have finished their obligatory duty; in the same way, we speak of people who have retired from public affairs. Therefore, we use the word "defunct" because the person in question has been deposed from life as [though] from a position, or because he has finished his last day on earth.

37. "Buried," *sepultus,* is so named because after death the body is without pulse or palpitation, that is, without motion. Sepulture is burial of the body: we say "inhume" or "bury"—this means to cover with earth.

3. PORTENTOUS MONSTERS

1. Varro says that portents are things which seem to have been born contrary to nature, but in truth, they are not contrary to nature, because they exist by the divine will, since the Creator's will is the nature of everything created. For this reason, the very pagans called God "Nature" sometimes, "god" at other times.

2. A portent, therefore, does not arise contrary to nature, but contrary to what nature is understood to be. Portents are also called "signs," "monstrosities," and "prodigies" because they seem to portend and to point out, to demonstrate, and the predict future happenings.

3. Portents, *portentum,* are named from portending, *portendere,* that is from "showing in advance," *praeostendere;* but signs, *ostentum,* [are so named] because they seem to point out some future event; prodigies, *prodigium,* are named because they "speak from afar," *porro dicere,* that is, they foretell the future. Monstrosities, *monstrum,* are named from an "admonition," *monitus,* because they point out something by signaling, or because they indicate what may immediately appear. This is the word's proper meaning, although it has been corrupted by the misuse of many writers.

4. Some portentous creations, however, seem to have been made as an indication of future events, since

---

2. 30: This passage suggests that the greatest curse of the aged is their feelings of being weak and burdensome to others, an observation of great insight.

2. 32: *Immaturus* is used, of death, at Servius *Aeneid* 6. 429 and 11. 28 as an agricultural term, meaning "unripe."

2. 33: Otto attributes this citation to Caesar the Grammarian.

2. 34: See also XX. 10 and Servius *Aeneid* 1. 731.

2. 35: There are fuller discussions of funerary matters and their related etymologies at Servius *Aeneid* 6. 481; 2. 539 and 11. 143; and at Varro, *De lingua latina* 5. 23 and 5. 166.

2. 37: *Cf.* Servius *Aeneid* 3. 42: *nam sepultus est quasi sine pulsu.*

3. 1: Augustine discusses portents at *De civitate Dei* 21. 8.

3. 2: *Cf.* Cicero, *De divinatione* 2: *quia enim ostendunt, portendunt, monstrant, praedicunt; ostenta, monstra, prodigia dicuntur.*

3. 3: See *Differentiarum* I. 457–459 [*PL* 83: 56–57]; Servius and Servius Daniel *Aeneid* 2. 681 and Servius *Aeneid* 3. 366.

3. 4: Lindsay's *creationes in sinificationibus* should certainly read *c. in significationibus.*

Tertullian, *De anima* 46. 3–12 [Waszink 63–65] reviews

God now and then wishes to tell of coming events through some fault or other in newborn creatures, as also through dreams and oracles, by which He warns and admonishes certain peoples or individuals of impending disaster: this is proved by abundant experience.

5. The birth of a vixen to a mare portended the destruction of Xerxes' kingdom. A monster was born of Alexander's wife which had human upper parts, which were dead, and the lower parts of various animals, which were living, indicating the king's sudden death, for the worse parts outlived the better. But these monsters which are sent as signs do not live very long, dying as soon as they are born.

6. There is a difference between a portent, *portentum*, and a prodigy, *portentuosum*, for portents are things which have been transformed, as it is reported that a woman in Umbria gave birth to a serpent. Whence Lucan [1. 563]: *matremque suus conterruit infans*, "and her infant terrifies the mother." But a prodigy undergoes a slight change, for example, as in being born with six fingers.

7. Prodigies or portents therefore exist either by virtue of some bodily size beyond the measure common among men, such as was Tityon who, stretched out, occupied nine acres of land, as Homer testifies; or else by a smallness of bodily stature, as the dwarfs or those whom the Greeks call Pygmies, because they are about a cubit tall. Others from a hugeness of parts, such as misshapen heads, or superfluous members, as two-headed or three-handed men, or the Cynodontes, a people with double rows of teeth.

8. Others stem from a lack of parts, among whom one part is very different from the other, as hand from hand, or foot from foot; or by reason of a cutting off, *decisio*, such as those who are begotten without a hand or a head, whom the Greeks call *steresios;* others are *praenumeria*, when only a head or a leg is born.

9. Others are transformed in part, such as those having the face of a lion or a dog, or a bull's head or body, as it is recalled that the Minotaur was born of

Pasiphaë. The Greeks call this *HETEROMORPHIA*. Others are transformed in every part into a portent of another kind of creature, such as the account that a calf was born of a woman. Others involve a change of position without transformation, such as eyes in the chest or the forehead, or ears above the temple, or such as Aristotle reports, an individual who had the liver on the left side and the spleen on the right.

10. Others [are portents] because of a certain growing together, such as those who have on one hand more fingers than is natural, all adhering together, and fewer on the other hand, or [with the same situation] in the feet; others are portentous because of an immature or disproportionate growth, such as those who are born with teeth or bearded or gray-haired; other are characterized by a complex of many differences, such as that multiformed monster which we spoke of above [§ 5] in connection with Alexander.

11. Some arise from a mixture of sex, as those which are called *ANDROGUNOI* or *HERMAPHRO-DITAI*. Hermaphrodites are so called because in them both sexes are manifest. *HERMÈS* among the Greeks means "masculine," *APHRODITÈ*, "feminine." These have the right breast of a man and the left of a woman and, after coitus in turn can both sire and bear children.

12. Just as among individual races there are certain members who are monsters, so also among mankind as a whole, certain races are monsters, like the giants, the Cynocephali, the Cyclopes and others.

13. The giants, *Gigantes*, are named from an etymology in the Greek language, for they think that they are *GÈGENEIS*, that is, "earth born," because the legend among them is that their mother, Earth, being of immense size, produced young like herself: "earth" is called *GÈ*, "born," *GENOS;* and in spite of the ordinary people calling them "sons of earth," their origin is uncertain.

14. Certain men, unversed in the Sacred Scriptures, think quite incorrectly that before the flood, apostate angels had intercourse with the daughters of men, and that from this were born the giants, that is, the very strong and large men by whom the earth was filled.

15. *Cynocephali* are so named because they have the heads of a dog, and by their barking prove that they are more beast than human. These arise in India.

---

various prophetic dreams which "came true," and it was common Stoic belief that dreams were sent to advise men; see also Lactantius, *De opificio Dei* 18 [*CSEL* 27: 59].

3. 7: Tityon, seen by Odysseus in Hades, covered nine acres of ground as two vultures tore at his liver (the seat of carnal lust) to punish his rape of Leto; see *Odyssey* 11. 576 ff. and Servius *Aeneid* 6. 596. Pygmies, in Greek legend, are dwarfs from Africa or India, which carry on warfare with cranes; see *Iliad* 3. 6. African pygmies still hunt cranes.

3. 9: The reference to the liver on the left side probably refers to a case of *situs inversus*, wherein the internal organs form a mirror image of their usual conformation. Although without adverse effect on the patient's well-being, it is difficult to imagine the source of this report (attributed to Aristotle, and unverified by this writer) except as an accidental finding on dissection of the body by an individual with enough experience to recognize it as an anomaly.

3. 11: On hermaphroditism, see Pliny 8. 2 and 11. 49; and Augustine, *De civitate Dei* 16. 8.

3. 13–14: Hesiod (*Theogonis* 185) relates that giants are the sons of Earth (Gê), born of the blood of heaven (Uranus) which fell to earth. Later accounts of battles between giants and gods in the Greek hero cycles were interpreted as conflicts between civilization and barbarism, or between good and evil. See also Augustine, *De civitate Dei* 3. 4.

3. 15: The legends of Cynocephali, from India, may be derived from the baboon or hyena: an allusion to the lowest Hindu castes is less likely, see Ctesias, *Indica* 23; and see also XII. 2. 32 and Augustine, *De civitate Dei* 16. 8.

16. The same India also produced the Cyclopes, so named because they are said to have one eye in the 'middle of their foreheads. They are also called *AGRIOPHAGITAI* because they eat only the flesh of wild animals.

17. It is believed that the *Blemmyae* in Libya are born as headless trunks, that they have both eyes and mouth in their chests; and that there are others, born without necks, having eyes in their shoulders.

18. The monstrous appearance of races in the Far East is described: some without noses, the face being entirely smooth, with shapeless countenance; others having an upper lip so prominent that when asleep they can cover their whole face against the sun's heat with it; others with frozen mouths, who suck gruel with an oat-straw through a little opening. Some are said to be without tongues, using nods and motions to speak with each other.

19. They say that the *Panotii* who are in Scythia have such huge ears that they cover their entire body with them: *PAN* in Greek is said for "all," *OTA*, "ears."

20. The *Artabatitae* in Ethiopia are reported to walk on all fours like beasts, and none of them passes the fortieth year of age.

21. Satyrs are little mannikins with hooked noses, horns in their foreheads and feet like those of goats such as the one Saint Antony saw in the desert, who also, questioned by this servant of God, is said to have replied, saying [Jerome, *Vita Pauli Eremitae* 8]: *Mortalis ego sum unus ex accolis heremi, quos vario delusa errore gentilitas Faunos Satyrosque colit,* "I am mortal—one of those inhabitants of the desert whom the pagans, deceived by various errors, worship as Fauns and Satyrs."

22. Some are also called forest-dwelling men, whom some call "fig-like Fauns."

23. The race of Sciopodes is said to exist in Ethiopia, with only one leg but marvelous speed withal: the Greeks call them *SKIOPODES* because in the summertime they stretch out on their backs, covering themselves with the shadows of their huge feet.

24. The Antipodes in Libya have their soles turned around behind their legs, and have eight toes on the soles.

---

3. 21: See also XII. 2. 33.

3. 22: *Ficarius,* "fig-like," perhaps from "fig-dwelling," which Lewis and Short refer to the satyr's lasciviousness. This seems to be a veiled reference to phallic worship, a problem for Christian leaders in and after Isidore's time. *Cf.* H. M. Westropp and C. S. Wake, *Influence of the phallic idea in the religions of antiquity* (2nd ed., New York, 1875), p. 85: "In Greece and Western Asia the favorite wood for the 'stocks' and phallic pillars, according to St. Clement of Alexandria, was the fig. The leaves of this tree, it will be remembered, were used in the garden of Eden; and the fruit has had a peculiar symbolical meaning for thousands of years."

25. The Hippopodes, having human form and horses' feet, are in Scythia.

26. It is said that there is a race standing twelve feet tall in India, called the *MAKROBIOI*. In the same country, there is also a race with a stature of one cubit, whom the Greeks call Pygmies, after the cubit, and of whom we have spoken above [§ 7]. These live in the mountains of India which are near the ocean.

27. It is reported that there is [also] in that same India a race whose women conceive when they are five years old, and who do not live past the age of eight.

28. Certain other fabled portents of men are written of which do not exist, but which have been invented to explain things such as Geryon, King of Spain, who is reported to have had three forms, because there were once three brothers having such perfect concord that it was as though one spirit existed in three bodies.

29. The Gorgons also were serpent-tressed courtesans who changed those who looked upon them into stones, having one eye which they used in turn. These were three sisters alike in one common beauty, as alike in the possession of a common appearance, which so stupefied their beholders that they were reputed to turn them into stones.

30. The story is that there were three Sirens, part maiden and part bird, having wings and claws, who made music—one with voice, one with the flute, and one on the lyre—and who pulled sailors, enchanted by their music, down to shipwreck.

31. Really though, they were harlots who went across the sea and, because they met with poverty, they pretended that it was caused by shipwreck; to have had wings and claws because love flies and inflicts wounds; and were said to have tarried on the waves because Venus came from the Deep.

32. Some say that Scylla was a woman girdled about with dogs' heads, surrounded by great barking, because in the strait of the Sicilian Sea, sailors terrified by the wavetops rushing at them thought that those waves the whirlpools of the devouring sea tossed against each other barked.

33. Some made up also certain irrational beings to be monsters, such as Cereberus, the Hound of Hell, having three heads, indicating through him the three ages which death devours, namely, infancy, youth and old age. Some, however, think that he was named Cereberus as though *KREOBOROS*, that is, "flesh-devouring."

34. And they say that the Hydra was a serpent with nine heads, which is called *excetra* in Latin, because as soon as one head was cut off, three grew up. The correct account is that Hydra was a place spewing forth

---

3. 29: See Servius *Aeneid* 2. 616 and Augustine, *De civitate Dei* 18. 13.

3. 32: Ovid, *Metamorphoses* 14. 73, also rationalizes this sea monster dwelling in a cave opposite Charybdis to a rock or some other menace to navigation.

water, destroying a neighboring city which, when one channel was closed off, many more burst open. Hercules, seeing this, dried the place up, and thus closed off the water's channel.

35. For *Hydra* is named from "water": Ambrose mentions this in a comparison with heresies, saying [*De fide* 1. 4] : *Haeresis enim velut quaedam hydra fabularum vulneribus suis crevit; et dum saepe reciditur, pullulavit igni debita incendioque peritura,* "Heresy is like a certain hydra in the fables, increasing by its very wounds, and while it often gives ground, again it bursts forth with its usual fire and consuming flames."

36. They have made the Chimaera out to be a three-formed beast: a lion's features, the hinder parts of a dragon, and the middle parts of a goat. Certain naturalists say that this was not an animal, but a mountain in Cilicia, nursing in some places lions and goats, burning in some and in other places full of serpents. Bellerophontes made this place inhabitable, whence he is said to have killed the Chimaera.

37. Centaurs are given their name from their appearance, that is, man mixed with horse, whom some say were Thessalonian knights, but because running about in battle they seemed to be one body of men and horses, they assert that Centaurs were thence invented.

38. The name of Minotaurs was taken from a bull and a man, such a beast as the fabulists say was shut in the Labyrinth, and concerning which Ovid says [*Ars Amoris* 2. 24] : *semibovemque virum, semivirumque bovem,* "A man half-bull, a bull half-man."

39. An ass-centaur, *onocentaurus,* is so named because it is said to have partly the appearance of man and partly ass; and likewise the Hippocentaurs, because the natures of horses and men are thought to be united in them.

4. TRANSFORMATIONS

1. Some monstrous transformations of men and changes into beasts are reported, such as that very famous enchantress Circe, who is said also to have changed Ulysses' companions into beasts; and the Arcadians who, selected by lot, swam across a certain pond and were straightway changed into wolves.

2. That the companions of Diomedes were changed into birds is proved, not by fabled fictions but by historical evidence. But some assert that witches can be made from human beings: the appearance of criminals is changed for much villany, and they are transformed into beasts, in every part of their bodies, whether by magic incantations or the poison of herbs.

3. Many beings even undergo transformations quite naturally, and having become debased from their original forms, are changed into various appearances; just as bees come from the decaying flesh of cattle, so also scarabs from horses, locusts from mules, and scorpions from crabs. Ovid writes [*Metamorphoses* 15. 369] :

> *Concava litorei si demas brachia cancri,*
> *scorpio exibit, caudaque minabitur unca.*

"If you take away the curved arms of the seashore crab, a scorpion will emerge and threaten with hooked tail."

---

4. 2: There is a reference to the use of magic in human transformations at Augustine, *De civitate Dei* 18. 16.

4. 3: References to the growth of swarms of bees from the carcasses of dead animals are common in ancient literature: see Judges 14: 8, for example, or Vergil, *Georgics* 4. 555–556. These two references, at least, can be explained by confusion between the bee (*Apis melifer*) and *Eristolis taenax*, which looks very much like the bee, but which deposits its eggs in carrion. Several species of *Scarabaediae* (*S. troginae* or *S. coprinae*, for example) live in dung or dry decomposing animal matter—the "locust" of Exodus was probably *Schistocerca gregaria*, whose eggs are placed singly in the soil. The morphology of the cray-fish, the common crab and well-known scavenger, is similar enough to the scorpion to cause confusion.

ISIDORE OF SEVILLE *ON MEDICINE*

A translation of

ISIDORI ETYMOLOGIARUM SIVE ORIGINUM LIBER IV:

De Medicina

1. MEDICINE

1. Medicine, *medicina,* is that which either protects or restores bodily health: its subject matter deals with diseases and wounds.

2. There pertain to medicine not only those things which display the skill of those to whom the name physician, *medicus,* is properly applied, but also food and drink, shelter and clothing. In short, it includes every defense and fortification by which our body is kept [safe] from external attacks and accidents.

2. ITS NAME

The name of medicine is thought to have been given it from "moderation," *modus,* that is, from a due proportion, which advises that things be done not to excess, but "little by little," *paulatim.* For nature is pained by surfeit but rejoices in moderation. Whence also those who take drugs and antidotes constantly, or to the point of saturation, are sorely vexed, for every immoderation brings not health but danger.

3. THE FOUNDERS OF MEDICINE

1. Among the Greeks, the discoverer and founder of the art of medicine is said to have been Apollo. His son, Aesculapius, added to it by his fame and works.

2. However, after Aesculapius died from a lightning bolt, it is said that the healing art was forbidden and that the art died along with its founder, and was hidden for nearly five hundred years, until the time of Artaxerxes, King of Persia. At that time, Hippocrates, born on the Island of Cos and whose father was Aesculapius, restored it to light.

4. THE THREE SECTS OF PHYSICIANS

1. These three men founded as many sects. The first, or Methodist, *Methodica,* was founded by Apollo, whose remedies are also discussed in poems. The second, or Empiric, *Enpirica,* that is, the most fully tested, was established by Aesculapius and is based upon observed factual experience alone, and not on mere signs and indications. The third, or Logical, *Logica,* that is, rational sect, was founded by Hippocrates.

2. For having discussed the qualities of the ages of life, regions and illnesses, Hippocrates thoroughly and rationally investigated the management of the art; diseases were searched through to their causes in the light of reason [and their cure was rationally studied]. The Empirics follow only experience; the Logical join reason to experience; the Methodists study the relationships of neither elements, times, ages, nor causes, but only the properties of the diseases themselves.

5. THE FOUR HUMORS OF THE BODY

1. Health, *sanitas,* consists in an integrity of the body and a harmonious proportion in its nature as regarding the hot and moist qualities embodied in the blood, wherefore it is called "health" as though the state of the blood, *sanguis.*

2. The word "disease," *morbus,* is a general term which includes all bodily afflictions; our elders called it "disease" to indicate by this name the power of death, *mors,* which could arise therefrom. Healing, *curatio,* consists in a middle course between health and disease for, unless congruent with the disease, it does not conduce to health.

3. All diseases arise from the four humors: that is, from blood and yellow bile, from black bile and phlegm. [Healthy people are maintained by them and the ill suffer from them. When any of the humors increase beyond the limits set by nature, they cause illnesses.]

---

1. 1: See note on IV. 9. 5–6 below, and *cf.* Pseudo-Soranus, *Quaestiones medicinales* 10 [Rose 248]: *medicina dicitur a medendo id est sanitatem praestando.*

3. 1: Pseudo-Soranus, *Quaestiones medicinales* Prooem. [Rose 243]: *Medicinam quidem invenit Apollo, amplicavit Aesculapius, perfecit Hippocrates.* At VIII. 11, 3, Aesculapius is mentioned as the founder of medicine, and at XIV. 6. 18, *Coos* is "an island near the province of Attica in which the physician Hippocrates was born."

3. 2: The traditional account (see, e.g., Vergil, *Aeneid* 7. 772–775) is that Aesculapius restored the murdered Hippolytus to life, and that, enraged that another should usurp his divine healing power, Jupiter killed Aesculapius with a lightning bolt.

4. 1: See note on IV. 9. 2 below, and Celsus, *De medi-*

cina Prooem. 9, for the three areas of post-classical medical practice. Does Isidore confuse *Asclepius* with *Aesculapius?*

5. 1: Fletcher, *op. cit.,* p. 92, states that in this chapter, Isidore's source is Galen, *Definitiones medicae,* but some Latin version such as the Pseudo-Soranus text published by Rose seems more probable.

5. 2: Schwarz suggests *quo [vocabulo] inde veteres* in place of *quod inde veteres,* but Lindsay's text is followed.

5. 3: There is a similar discussion of humoral factors in the production of disease, with the qualification that acute diseases are accompanied by a fever and that chronic diseases have little or no fever at Aurelius, *De acutis passionibus,* Prooem. [Daremberg 479]. Pseudo-Soranus, *Quaestiones medicinales* 85–86 [Rose 257] gives a briefer definition with examples of specific disease types, and there is a more extended account at Galen, *Definitiones medicae* [Kühn 19: 387].

Just as there are four elements, so also there are four humors, and each humor imitates its own proper element: blood the air; yellow bile fire; black bile earth; and phlegm water. Thus, there are four humors as well as four elements which preserve our bodies.

4. Blood, *sanguis*, derives its name from a Greek etymology, because it grows and sustains and lives. The Greeks call yellow bile [such] because it is bounded by the space of one day, whence also it is called *choler*, that is, *fellicula*, for this is an effusion of bile, *fellis effusio*. For the Greeks call bile *CHOLĒ*.

5. Black bile, *melancholia*, is so named because it is a mixture of the dregs from black blood with an abundance of bile: the Greeks call "black," *MELAS* and "bile," *CHOLĒ*.

6. Blood, *sanguis*, is named in Latin because it is pleasant to the taste, *suavis;* whence also men in whom the humor blood predominates are pleasant and agreeable.

7. Phlegm, *phlegma*, however, is named because it is cold, for the Greeks call coldness *PHLEGMONĒ*. By these four humors healthy people are maintained and the ill suffer from them, for when they increase beyond the limits set by nature, they cause illnesses. The acute diseases, which the Greeks call *OXEA*, arise from blood and yellow bile, but the longstanding disorders, which the Greeks call *CHRONIA*, come from phlegm and black bile.

6. ACUTE DISEASES

1. *OXEIA* is [the name applied to] an acute disease which either passes away quickly or kills speedily, such as pleurisy, phrenitis. The word for "acute" in Greek is *OXUS*, which means "rapid." *CHRONIA* is [the name applied to] a protracted disease of the body which tarries for long periods of time, such as gout, phthisis. Among the Greeks, *CHRONOS* is said for "time." Certain diseases, however, are named after their own proper causes.

2. Fever, *febris*, is named from "boiling," *fervor*, for it is an abundance of heat.

---

5. 4: See Caelius Aurelianus, *De morbis acutis* 3. 19.
5. 5: Galenic physiology generally held that the yellow bile was separated from the blood of the portal vein, passing to the gall bladder and thence to the duodenum. The heavy impurity, the black bile, passed to the spleen. Phlegm was often the residue of digested food.
5. 6: See XI. 1. 122.
5. 7: *PHLEGMA* is the word for fire, heat or flame and, by derivation, for inflammation in the medical sense, but may stand for the humor phlegm. *PHLEGMONĒ* does not seem to have been used for *rigor*, "coldness" or "stiffness," but for inflammation. See IV. 6. 7.
OXEA is an Ionic form for *OXEIA*, the feminine form of *OXUS:* at I. 19. 1, *OXEIA* refers to the acute accent in Greek grammar. *CHRONIA* is the neuter plural of *CHRONIOS*, and is apparently an adverbial substantive.

3. *Frenesis* is named either from a hinderance of the mind, for the Greeks call the mind *PHRENES*, or because [those suffering this disease] gnash their teeth, for to gnash, *frendere*, is to strike the teeth together. It is a confusion accompanied by agitation and dementia, caused by the force of yellow bile.

4. *Cardia[ca]* [disease] derives its name from the heart, *cor*, because this is affected by any fear or pain, and the Greeks call the heart *KARDIA*. For it is a pain of the *cardia* accompanied by formidable apprehension.

5. *Lethargia* is named from "sleep": it is a catalepsy of the brain, *oppressio cerebri*, accompanied by forgetfulness and constant sleep as though of one snoring.

6. A sore throat, *synanche*, is named from constriction of the vital spirit and suffocation, for the Greeks

---

6. 3: See Appendix B, "Frenesis."
6. 4: *KARDIA* refers to the heart and precordium, but the word is often used with reference to the stomach. Galen and some other physicians located the "cardiac disease," *KARDIAKOS NOUSOS*, at the gastro-esophageal junction, almost precluding precise translation of the word: in this passage, *cordis passio* is untranslatable. At Celsus, *De medicina* 3. 19. 1, *cardiacus morbus* is collapse or syncope in general, and not *per se* disease of the heart or stomach. Isidore's "cardiac disease" is nothing more exact than the precordial and epigastric pain of many forms of biliary, cardio-pulmonary and gastro-intestinal disease. Caelius Aurelianus, *De morbis acutis* 2. 30–39, reviews some of the ancient ideas on cardiac disease, and there is a full differential diagnosis at Aurelius, *De acutis passionibus* 13 [Daremberg 710–713]. Francis Adams reviews this subject in his *The Seven Books of Paulus Aegineta* (London, 1844–1847) 1: pp. 292–296.
Cassius Felix, *De medicina* 64 [Rose 156–157] describes what must be acute myocardial failure with sweating, vomiting, fever, and joint pain.
6. 5: *Lethargia* does not seem to be encephalitis lethargica, but any comatose state, whether the result of infection, trauma, or toxin: any violent bodily insult can disrupt the respiration, and the terminal stages of illnesses marked by deep coma are often accompanied by snoring respiration. See Caelius Aurelianus, *De morbis acutis* 1. 40.
What ancient physicians called catalepsy, phrenitis, and lethargy were epidemic fevers whose identification is now conjectural in most cases, but which were marked by coma during their course or termination. They do not refer only to infection of the cerebral substance or meninges, and these terms must not be interpreted in their modern sense. Isidore seems to have something in mind akin to Aurelius, *De acutis passionibus* Prooem. [Daremberg 481]: *litarcos: oblivio quidem et somni juges, sed non necessario profundus est*, which suggests variable degrees of coma. Pseudo-Soranus, *Quaestiones medicinales* 12 [Rose 268] mentions meningeal tumor and cerebral abscess among possible causes of lethargy. See also Galen, *Definitiones medicae* 235 [Kühn 19: 413], Cassius Felix, *De medicina* 63 [Rose 155] and Caelius Aurelianus, *De morbis acutis* 2. 1–9.
6. 6: Isidore's *synanche* refers only to a painful sore throat which may progress to suffocation, whether it be from diphtheria, laryngeal edema or malignant disease. See also Paulus Aegineta, *Epitome* 3. 27; Aurelius, *De acutis passionibus* 12 [Daremberg 706]; Pseudo-Soranus, *Quaestiones medicinales* 202 [Rose 268] and Caelius Aurelianus, *De morbis acutis* 3. 1. 2.

say *SUNANCHEIN* for "to constrict." Those who suffer from this malady are strangled by pain of the pharynx.

7. *Fleumon* is a burning of the stomach with swelling and pain [or *PHLEGMONÊ* is restlessness with redness, pain, tension, hardness and a terrible swelling]. If such characterizes the onset, a fever follows, whence also is said *PHLEGMONÊ, APO PHLEGEI,* that is, "burning," *inflammare.* It derives its name from the feeling it evokes.

8. Pleurisy, *pleurisis,* is a sharp pain of the side accompanied by a fever and a bloody sputum: in Greek, the side is called *PLEURA,* whence [also] the pleuritic disease derives its name.

9. Pneumonia, *peripleumonia,* is a disease of the lung marked by sharp pain and a sighing respiration. The Greeks call the lung *PLEUMÔN,* whence also this disease is named.

10. Apoplexy, *apoplexia,* is a sudden effusion of blood by which those who die are suffocated. It is called apoplexy because it is caused by a sudden lethal blow. The Greeks call a blow *APOPLÊXIS.*

11. A cramp, *spasmus,* in Latin, is a sudden contraction of the bodily parts or tendons with a very sharp pain. They say that this disease is named after the heart, which is the principal source of our strength. It arises in two ways, from repletion or from inanition.

12. A stiff neck, *tetanus major,* is a contraction of tendons from the neck to the back.

13. A stitch in the side, *telum,* is a pain in the side. It is so named by the physicians since the body is transfixed by pain as though by a sword.

14. Colic, *ileos,* is an intestinal pain: whence also it is called *ilia.* The Greeks say "to muffle up" is †*ilios*†, be-

cause the intestines fold themselves in from the pain. These diseases are also called "the gripes," *turminosi,* from "torment of the intestines."

15. *HUDROPHOBIA,* that is, fear of water, for the Greeks call water *HUDÔR,* fear *PHOBOS,* whence also considering this fear of water, the Latins called this disease "madness," *lymphaticus.* It arises [either] from the bite of a rabid dog, or from spume falling from the air to the ground. Should man or beast touch this, he straightway becomes demented or is also made rabid.

16. A carbuncle, *carbunculus,* is named because in the beginning it is red like fire and in the end, black like a dead coal, *carbo extinctus.*

17. Plague, *pestilentia,* is a contagion which, when it takes hold of one person, quickly spreads to many. It arises from corrupt air, *corrupto aëre,* and by penetrating into the viscera settles there. Even though this disease often springs up from air-borne potencies, *per aërias potestates,* nevertheless it can never come about without the will of Almighty God.

18. It is termed "pestilence" as though a "little pasture," *pastulentia,* or because it feeds like a fire, as Vergil [*Aeneid* 5. 683]: *Toto descendit corpora pestis,* "The plague fell upon the whole body." Likewise, it is called "contagion," *contagium,* from "touch," *contingere,* for whomsoever it touches, it infects. It is also called *inguina* because it attacks the groins, *inguen.*

19. The same disease is also called *lues,* from "destruction" and "grief," *luctus,* since its course is so acute and rapid that one does not have enough time in which even to hope for life or for death, but a feeling of faintness comes on suddenly, bringing death at the same time.

7. CHRONIC DISEASES

1. *Chronia* is a protracted disease which tarries for long periods of time, such as gout, phthisis, for *CHRONOS* is said in Greek for "time."

2. Headache, *cephalea,* is named from its cause: it is a pain of the head, and the Greeks called the head *KEPHALÊ.*

6. 7: *Fleumon* might also be translated as "distension of the stomach," and the bracketed passage following rejected as an interpolation.

6. 8: See Scribonius Largus, *Conpositiones* 94: *qui lateris dolorem cum febre sentiunt, quos Graeci PLEURITIKOUS vocant.*

6. 10: If *apoplexia* here refers to cerebral hemorrhage or thrombosis, the English "stroke," this passage reflects ancient knowledge that paralysis and death from respiratory failure can follow such cerebral accidents. The Greek word refers to this and not to a sudden pulmonary hemorrhage, a much less likely alternative interpretation of this passage. Galen, *Definitiones medicae* 254 [Kühn 19: 415] clearly refers to coma and paralysis as characteristic of *apoplexia,* and see also Aurelius, *De acutis passionibus* 19 [Daremberg 720]; Cassius Felix, *De medicina* 65 [Rose 158] and Caelius Aurelianus, *De morbis acutis* 3. 5.

6. 11–12: At Caelius Aurelianus, *De morbis chronicis* 2. 63–64, *spasmos* is a functional nervous tic or muscular cramp. See also Galen, *Definitiones medicae* 236–239 [Kühn 19: 413–414] for definitions of *convulsio, tetanus, emprosthotonos,* and *ophisthotonos* in substantially their modern meanings, and their slightly differing form in Pseudo-Soranus, *Quaestiones medicinales* 203–206 [Rose 268]. Scribonius Largus, *Conpositiones* 101 associates tetanus especially with the contusions and lacerations suffered by gladiators in the arena.

6. 14: See Appendix C, "The Iliac Passion."

6. 15: There is a good account of rabies at Caelius Aurelianus, *De morbis acutis* 3. 9. 11, and Isidore's account resembles that at Aurelius, *De acutis passionibus* 21 [Daremberg 723–724], which includes a suggestion that reactions to rabid animals may be hysterical.

6. 16: Cassius Felix, *De medicina* 22 [Rose 37–38] ascribes carbuncles to a collection of hot blood and black bile, and *cf.* Scribonius Largus, *Conpositiones* 25: *carbunculos, quos ANTHRAKAS dicunt.*

6. 17–19: See Appendix D, "A Note on the Plague."

7. 2: In later Latin, *cephalgia* generally refers to an acute headache, and *cephalea* to a chronic headache. At Celsus, *De medicina* 4. 2. 2, *KEPHALAIA* is the chronic headache of malaria, endemic in the Mediterranean lowlands throughout the classical period.

3. Dimness of vision, *scothomia*, derives its name from its symptoms, because sudden shadows press upon the eyes, accompanied by a spinning of the head. We speak of *vertigo*, however, whenever it seems as though a wind were arising which sends the earth around in a circle.

4. In the same manner, the air-passages and blood vessels at the top of a man's head become inflated from the moisture resolved there, and produces gyrations before the eyes, whence also *vertigo* is named.

5. Epilepsy, *epilemsia*, is named because hanging over the mind, it equally also possesses the body. The Greeks term anything "weighing upon" *EPILÊPSIA*. It arises whenever the black bile happens to develop in excess and is turned in its course to the brain. This disease is also called the "falling sickness," *caduca*, because the sick man, falling down, *cadens*, suffers convulsions.

6. These the common people call "lunatics" since under the influence of the moon's cycle, *lunae cursus*, the snare of demons snatches them up. This likewise accounts for the term "ghost-ridden," *larvaticus*. It is the same thing as the comitial disease, that is, a greater and divine disease by which those who have fallen to the ground are held—it is powerful enough to make a strong man fall down and froth at the mouth.

7. It is called the comitial disease because if, among the pagans, this seized anyone on a meeting day set for the Comitia, this assembly was dismissed. However, there was a solemn day for the meeting of the Comitia at Rome on the kalends of January.

8. *Mania* is named from "insanity" or "fury," because the ancient Greeks called fury *MANIKÊ*, either from "unpropitiousness," *iniquitas*, which the Greeks called †*maniet* or from "divination," because the Greeks say *MANEIN* for to "divine."

9. *Melancholia* is named from black bile: the Greeks call black *MELAS*, and bile *CHOLÊ*. Epilepsy arises in the phantasy; melancholia in the reason; mania in the memory.

10. Intermittent fevers, *typi*, are chilling fevers incorrectly called *tipi* after a certain herb which grows in water. In Latin, "form and state," *forma atque status* are said for the disease is an accession and recession of the fever which recurs over regular intervals of time.

11. *Reuma*, in Greek, is called an "eruption" or a "flux" in Latin. Catarrh, *catarrhus*, is a continuous flow of rheum from the nostrils which, if it spreads to the pharynx, is called *BRANCHOS;* if to the thorax or lung, *PTUSIS.*

12. *Coryza* is a continuous flow from the head to the bones of the nostrils, and causes much annoyance from sneezing, whence also it gets the name *coryza*.

13. Hoarseness, *branchos*, is a constriction of the throat by a cold humor: the Greeks call the throat *BRANCHOS;* the pharynx, *fauces*, surrounds this region which we incorrectly term *branciae*.

14. Laryngitis, *raucedo*, is loss of the voice. This is also called *arteriasis*, because the voice is made hoarse and weak by any injury to the windpipe. Asthma, *suspirium*, derives its name because it is a difficulty in breathing, which the Greeks call *DUSPNOIA*, that is, a "suffocation," *praefocatio*.

15. Pneumonia, *peripleumonia*, gets its name from the lungs, since it is a swelling, *tumor*, of the lung marked by an effusion of blood-stained sputum.

16. Hemoptysis, *haemoptois*, [is] an emission of blood through the mouth, whence also it derives its name, because *HAIMA* is said for blood.

---

7. 3: Isidore differentiates between *scotomata* and *vertigo*, which Aurelius, *De acutis passionibus*, Prooem. [Daremberg 479] incorrectly equates. See also Caelius Aurelianus, *De morbis chronicis* 1. 4.

7. 5–7: Ancient medical thought generally assigned the moon a part in controlling epileptic attacks; see Owsei Temkin, *The Falling Sickness* (Baltimore, 1945), who quotes Isidore at p. 94, and for typical accounts of epileptic attacks, see Cassius Felix, *De medicina* 71 [Rose 168] and Pseudo-Soranus, *Quaestiones medicinales* 207 [Rose 268].

7. 8: Tertullian considered insanity primarily a disease of the soul rather than the mind; see his *De anima* 18. 9 [Waszink 25–26].

7. 9: This classification of psychiatric disturbances agrees with post-classical views on cerebral localization. Francis Adams (Paulus Aegineta, *op. cit.*, 1: p. 90) notes: "The later Greek authorities, as, for example, Theophilus Protospatharius and Nemesius, adopt a division of the brain as regards its connexion with mind, to which Galen and his immediate followers appear to have been strangers. According to it, fantasy is connected with the anterior part of the brain; cogitation, or the *discursus mentis*, with the middle; and memory with the posterior."

Isidore derives the word "bad," *malus*, from (X. 176) the word for black bile, concluding, "for this reason, those men are called melancholy who flee from human society and suspect even their dearest friends." (It is likely that many people now considered "nervous" would, in ancient times, have been classified as "melancholy.") Mental deficiency is briefly mentioned (X. 79) by Isidore: "Demented, *demens*, means the same thing as 'mindless,' *amens*, that is, without a mind, or indicates that such have diminished mental power. Foolish, *desipiens*, in that they begin to understand less than was their wont."

On the cerebral ventricles, see Augustine, *De Genesi ad litteram* 7. 18 [PL 34: 364].

7. 10: See Appendix E, "A Note on Undulant Fevers."

7. 14: *DUSPNOIA* means "difficulty in breathing," *ASTHMA* (from *AÔ*, "to blow") really means "short of breath" or perhaps "panting." What is here translated as *asthma* is the Latin *suspirium* which seems to refer to a variety of diseases, including bronchial and cardiac asthma, in which expiration is sometimes more difficult than inspiration. Caelius Aurelianus, *De morbis chronicis* 3. 1, distinguishes this from *orthopnea*, which he considers more serious. There is a discussion of the *morbus arteriacus* at Paulus Aegineta, *Epitome* 3. 28, but the ancient views are well summarized by Cassius Felix, *De medicina* 41 [Rose 93–94]: *asthma* is puffing or difficult breathing, *dyspnea* can refer to any respiratory difficulty and *orthopnea* is a feeling of suffocation when the patient lies flat.

7. 15: For descriptions of pneumonia, see Aurelius, *De acutis passionibus* 11 [Daremberg 705–706] and Caelius Aurelianus, *De morbis acutis* 2. 25–29.

17. *Tisis* is an ulceration and swelling in the lungs, which arises with greater facility in young people. It is called *PHTHISIS* among the Greeks because it is a consumption of the entire body.

18. Cough, *tussis,* is named in Greek from "depth," since it comes from the depths of the chest: the contrary of this is high up in the throat, where the uvula tickles.

19. An abscess, *apostoma,* gets its name from "collection," for the Greeks call a collection *apostoma.*

20. Empyema, *enpiis,* is named from an internal abscess, either in the side or in the abdomen, accompanied by pain, fever, coughing, and an abundant purulent sputum.

21. Hepatic disease, *hepaticus morbus,* is so named since it is an affection of the liver, for the Greeks call the liver *HÊPAR.*

22. *Lienosis* takes its name from the spleen, for the Greeks say *SPLÊN* for "spleen."

23. Dropsy, *hydropis,* takes its name from a watery humor of the skin, for the Greeks call water *HUDÔR.* It is a subcutaneous accumulation of fluid, marked by a turgid swelling and a fetid, labored breath.

24. Nephritis, *nefresis,* receives its name from weakness of the kidneys, for the Greeks call the kidneys *NEPHROI.*

25. Paralysis, *paralesis,* is named from a destruction, *inpensatio,* of the body brought about by much cooling of the body, either as a whole or in part.

26. Cachexia, *cacexia,* takes its name from injury to [or the habitus of] the body: the Greeks have called a troublesome vexation *KACHEXIA.* This disease arises from the patient's intemperance, or from inept treatment with drugs, or marks a slow recovery from disease.

27. Atrophy, *atrofia,* gets its name from a shrinking of the body, for the Greeks term cessation of nourishment *ATROPHIA.* It is a thinness of the body brought about by obscure causes and [among those] convalescing little by little.

28. Obesity, *sarcia,* is a superfluous increment of flesh by which bodies are fattened beyond measure, for the Greeks call flesh *SARX.*

29. Sciatica, *sciasis,* is named after the part of the body which it attacks, for the Greeks call the bones of the joints upon whose highest points the heads of the thigh bones terminate, the *ISCHIA.* It arises whenever the phlegm descends into the straight bones and forms a contraction there.

30. The Greeks named gout, *podagra,* from the associated retraction of the feet and from the deadly pain, for we call everything which is cruel "rough," *agrestis,* abusively.

31. Arthritis, *artriticus morbus,* took its name from pain of the joints.

32. Calculus, *cauculus,* is a stone which arises in the bladder, whence also it is named: however, [the stone] is composed of phlegmatic matter.

33. Strangury, *stranguria,* is named because it draws together, *stringere,* [to produce] difficulty of urination.

34. *Satiriasis* is a continuous desire for venery marked by an erection of the natural parts: it is named after the Satyrs.

35. Diarrhea, *diarria,* is a continuous flow from the bowel not accompanied by vomiting.

36. Dysentery, *disinteria,* is a breach in the continuity, that is, an ulceration of the intestine, for *dis* is a division, *intera,* the intestine. It arises following a flux, which the Greeks call *DIARROIA.*

---

7. 17: *Tisis* is probably a corruption of *phthisis,* which it is unsafe to identify with pulmonary tuberculosis in all cases. See also Caelius Aurelianus, *De morbis chronicis* 2. 14 and *De morbis acutis* 2. 26.

7. 18: At Cassius Felix, *De medicina* 23 [Rose 68], *tussis* is a productive cough.

7. 19: *Collectio* is a later term than *abscessus; cf.* English, "a gathering."

7. 20: The description is compatible with an intra-abdominal abscess if the diaphragm is involved.

7. 23: In ancient medical writers generally, dropsy included ascites and anasarca, and Celsus distinguishes between three varieties of dropsy: ascites, anasarca, and tympanites. See also Caelius Aurelianus, *De morbis chronicis* 3. 8.

7. 24: Arevalo notes *nephritis, quae etiam DIABÊTÊS:* perhaps the polyuria was interpreted as a weakness of the kidneys.

7. 25: *Corporis inpensatio* suggests an extensive disorder interfering with sensation, coordination, and other bodily functions. There is a long description of such a state at Cassius Felix, *De medicina* 54 [Rose 139–140].

7. 26: See Celsus, *De medicina* 2. 1. 22; Caelius Aurelianus, *De morbis chronicis* 3. 6; and Pseudo-Soranus, *Quaestiones medicinales* 199 [Rose 267–268].

7. 27: For discussions of *atrophia,* see Caelius Aurelianus, *De morbis chronicis* 2. 14 and 3. 7.

7. 28: Some manuscripts read *sarcoma* in place of *sarcia,* "obesity," which the verb *saginare,* "to fatten," requires.

7. 29: See Cassius Felix, *De medicina* 53 [Rose 137] and Caelius Aurelianus, *De morbis chronicis* 5. 1.

7. 30: See Caelius Aurelianus, *De morbis chronicis* 5. 2.

7. 35–36: In ancient nosology generally, diarrhea is looseness of the bowels with frequent but relatively painless passage of watery stools; dysentery is painful, prostrating, and often marked by the passage of blood from mucosal ulceration. Typhoid fever, various parasitic infestations, and colonic malignancy were doubtless lumped together with the dysenteries. Aurelius describes *diarria* as above, but notes that it may be followed after some days by dysentery: *De acutis passionibus* 15 [Daremberg 717].

The ancient *cholera* was an entity now difficult to identify: Aurelius (*De acutis passionibus* 14 [Daremberg 715]) notes that it is accompanied by diarrhea, nausea, vomiting, and prostration. Colic was distinguished by swelling and pain of the viscus; see Cassius Felix, *De medicina* 51 [Rose 130–131], and see Appendix C, "The Iliac Passion." Caelius Aurelianus has a somewhat different point of view, and he considers diarrhea an acute, dysentery a chronic, disease; see his *De morbis acutis* 3. 19–22 and *De morbis chronicis* 4. 6.

37. *Lienteria* is named because it causes food to pass through the soft parts of the intestines as though there were nothing in the way.

38. The colic disease, *colica*, is named after the intestine which the Greeks call the *KÓLON*.

39. *Ragadiae* are named because they are fissures or wrinkles gathered around orifices. These are also called hemorrhoids, *emorroida*, from the flow of blood, since the Greeks call blood *HAIMA*.

8. DISEASES WHICH APPEAR ON THE BODY'S SURFACE

1. Mange, *alopicia* is a loss of the hair in patches circumscribed by reddish-yellow hairs having the color of copper, called by this name from a resemblance to the animal, the fox, which the Greeks call *ALÓPĚX*.

2. Parotitis, *parotida*, is hardness or abscesses near the ears which arise from fevers or any other [cause], whence they are called *PARÓTIS*, for the Greeks call the external ears *ÓTA*.

3. Freckles, *lentigo*, are little spotted marks, round in shape, named after a species of lentil, *lenticula*.

4. Erysipelas, *erisipela*, is that [disease] which the Latins call "the sacred fire," indicating by the use of a word in a sense opposite its proper meaning that it is an abominable disease. The skin of those affected grows red on the surface with a fiery redness; then, the redness having subsided, the disease progresses as though nearby places were invaded by fire so that a fever arises in addition.

---

7. 37: *Lienteria* seems to have been something akin to sprue or celiac disease, in which failure of digestion and absorption causes the patient to pass bulky, fatty stools sometimes containing undigested food as he becomes progressively more malnourished, succumbing eventually to infection or inanition. At Celsus, *De medicina* 4. 19. 1, and Aretaeus, *De morbis chronicis* 2. 7, it is probably a high gastro-intestinal obstruction. Paulus Aegineta, *Epitome* 3. 40, describes two varieties of lientery: one arises from superficial intestinal ulceration or scarring following dysentery, and another develops from "atony" of the bowel, apparently related to celiac disease or tropical sprue. Passage of food, in lientery, is rapid, subjective feelings of distress are intense and the food passed from the anus may appear almost unchanged. Cassius Felix, *De medicina* 48 [Rose 124] has about the same process in mind when he describes lientery.

7. 39: *Ragada* refers to fissures or ulcerations near the anus, the commonest being an infected pilonidal sinus, not to hemorrhoids. *Cf.* Scribonius Largus, *Conpositiones* 223: *fissuras ani diutinas, quas RHAGADAS dicunt,* and see Cassius Felix, *De medicina* 74 [Rose 178].

8. 1: Ancient folklore held that the vegetation upon which a fox urinated was forthwith killed, leaving burnt patches, and this is often suggested as the origin of the word *alopecia,* "fox mange." See Cassius Felix, *De medicina* 5 [Rose 12] and Pseudo-Soranus, *Quaestiones medicinales* 217 [Rose 269].

8. 2: Apparently endemic mumps; see Paulus Aegineta, *Epitome* 3. 23 for discussions of endemic and epidemic mumps.

5. Herpes, *serpedo,* is a redness of the skin accompanied by prominent pustules, and takes its name from "creeping," *serpere,* because it creeps gradually along the members.

6. Impetigo, *inpetigo,* is a dry scab elevated from the body, rough and round in shape: the common people call this *sarna.*

7. Pruritis, *prurigo,* is named from its itching, *perurere,* and burning.

8. Nyctalopia, *nyctalmos,* is a disease whereby vision is taken away by day even though the eyes be open, and is restored as the shadows of night begin to fall, or vice versa, as many prefer to have it, sight being restored by day and lost by night.

9. Warts, *verruca,* are one thing, *satiriasis* another. Warts occur singly, but in *satiriasis,* more than one [lesion] is present, and more are discovered around the first.

10. *Scabies* and *lepra:* each disease is marked by roughness of the skin, with itching and scaling, but the roughness and scaling in scabies is finer textured. It gets its name as though it cast off these scales like off-scourings, for SCABIES [sounds] as though SQUAMIES, "scales."

11. *Lepra,* on the other hand, is a scaly roughness of the skin, resembling the herb garden-cress, *lepida,* whence it takes its name, its color turns now black, now white, now red. *Lepra* is recognized in the human body as follows: if among the healthy parts of the skin there appears a different color scattered variously, or if this color spreads everywhere so much that it makes everything of one, but changed, color.

12. The disease *elefantiacus* is named from its similarity to the elephant, the skin of which is naturally hard and rough, and the name has been given to the disease among human beings because the surface of the body becomes similar to the skin of elephants, or

---

8. 5: This seems to be herpes zoster; *cf.* Scribonius Largus, *Conpositiones* 247: *zonam, quam Graeci HERPĒTA dicunt.*

8. 6: See Cassius Felix, *De medicina* 11 [Rose 19].

8. 8: The variant *qua per diem* is translated in place of Lindsay's *quae per diem.*
Nyctalopia, caused by congenital absence of the retinal rods or cones, can take the form of day or night blindness as the case may be. See Paulus Aegineta, *Epitome* 3. 22 and Scribonius Largus, *Conpositiones* 99.

8. 9: Probably *pityriasis* should be read in place of *satiriasis,* discussed at IV. 7. 34; see W. D. Sharpe, "A suggested emendation of Isidore of Seville, *Etymologiae* 4. 8. 9," *Traditio* 14 (1958): 377–378.

8. 10–11: See Leviticus 13: 1–6.

8. 12: This *elefanticus morbus* refers to a cutaneous infection of some kind, and not to any of the modern diseases called elephantiasis. That due to lymphedema was called *elephantiasis Arabum;* *elephantiasis Graecorum* in *Plinii Secundi Iunioris de medicina* (ed. Valentine Rose [Leipzig, 1875], p. 33) is a cutaneous infection spreading from one nidus. See also Cassius Felix, *De medicina* 73 [Rose 175].

because the pain is immense, like the animal itself from which its name has been taken.

13. Jaundice, *hicteris*, the Greeks have named after a certain animal because it has the color of yellow bile. The Latins term this the arcuate disease, from its resemblance to the rainbow, but Varro says that this disease is "gold-bearing," *auriginis*, because of its golden color. Some think that the same disease is termed that of kings in that it is the more readily cured by a regimen of good wines and rich foods.

14. *Cancer* is named from its resemblance to a certain marine animal: physicians say that it is a wound which admits of cure by no medications, and for this reason they usually cut off the member in which cancer has arisen from the body, so that [the patient] may live a little longer. In truth, yet death will come from it, although a little later.

15. A furuncle, *furunculus*, is a swelling rising to a point, named because it burns, as though a little coal, *fervunculus*, whence also in Greek it is called *ANTHRAX*, which means "fiery."

16. A stye, *ordeolus*, is a very small purulent abscess in the hairs of the eyelids, wide in the middle and extending on either end much like a grain of barley, *hordeum*, whence is derived its name.

17. *Oscedo* is that by which infants' mouths are ulcerated, named from their sluggishness in opening their mouths.

18. *Frenusculus* [refers to] ulcers around the margins of the mouth, similar to those in beasts of burden from chafing at the bit.

19. Ulcer, *ulcus*, [means] the same as festering. Wound, *vulnus*, [is an injury] made by iron, as though by force, *vis*. And ulcer because it smells like an olive, *olcus*, whence also "ulcer," *ulcera*.

20. A pustule, *pustula*, is a swelling on the surface of the skin, like an abscess.

21. A papule, *papula*, is a very small elevation of the skin surrounded by redness, and that is why it is called PAPULA, which sounds like PUPULA, "pupil" [of the eye].

22. Fistula, *syringio* [. . .] Bloody-matter, *sanies*, is named because it arises from blood. For blood is changed into bloody-matter by heat generated by the wound. Bloody-matter does not arise in any place unless blood is present, since nothing can putrefy unless, like blood, it is hot and moist. Bloody-matter and decomposition, *tabes*, differ from one another, for, although a discharge of bloody-matter is [a mark] of the living, decomposition [is a mark] of the moribund.

23. A scar, *cicatrix*, is a covering of a wound, which preserves the natural color of the parts, named because it draws wounds together and covers them.

9. REMEDIES AND MEDICATIONS

1. The healing of medicine is not to be despised, for we also recall that Isaiah ordered a certain medication for Ezechiel when he was ill, and the Apostle Paul said that Timothy ought to take a little wine.

2. The healing of disease is, however, of three sorts: pharmaceutical, which the Latins call "medications"; surgical, which the Latins call "operations using the hands," for hand is called *CHEIR* in Greek; and dietetic, which the Latins call "a rule," for it is careful attention to the laws of [daily] living. There are three species of cure, taken as a whole: the first group is dietetic, the second pharmaceutical, and the third surgical.

3. Dietetic consists in an observation of the laws of living; pharmacy is a cure using medicaments. Surgery is an incision using iron instruments, since those conditions not responding to treatment with drugs are excised with iron.

4. In more ancient times, medicine consisted entirely in herbs and juices: methods of treatment began in such manner, later with iron [instruments] and other medications.

---

8. 14: Cancer of the female breast was well known in ancient times; see, e.g., Augustine, *De civitate dei* 22. 8. 3 and Scribonius Largus, *Conpositiones* 102.

8. 15: This is a very vague description which is probably not of modern *anthrax*, not particularly painful, nor can the ancient *anthrax* be safely identified with smallpox or measles. Francis Adams (Paulus Aegineta, *op. cit.*, 1: pp. 330–335) reviews the problem.

8. 17: Adams, in a note on Paulus Aegineta, *Epitome* 1. 10, identifies *oscedo*, in Isidore, with aphthous stomatitis.

8. 19: The distinction between *ulcus* and *vulnus* in Isidore's account is an important one. According to Adams, *The genuine works of Hippocrates* (London, 1849) 1: 68, the word *HELKOS* meant "both a wound inflected by an external body and a solution of [bodily] continuity from any internal disease." By Isidore's time, *vulnus* is the former and *ulcus* the latter.

8. 22: *Syringa* is used synonymously with *syrinx*, *SURINX*, or fistula; Schwarz suggests *syringio*, Otto *SURINGION*. This is probably a lemma word left undefined by Isidore and his editor, and can refer to any fistulous or sinus tract.

Ancient medical writers generally accepted the theory that pus was derived from the blood; cf. Hippocrates, *On ulcers* 1: "A sore suppurates when the blood is changed and becomes heated; so that becoming putrid, it constitutes the pus of such ulcers." *Sanies* has a more general meaning of "diseased blood" and *tabes* can refer to any gradual wasting process; used in Isidore's sense, *tabes* seems to refer to any necrosis or gangrene. See Celsus, *De medicina* 5. 26. 20 for an account of various types of pus.

8. 23: As in Isidore, at Scribonius Largus, *Conpositiones* 241, cicatrix refers not only to a scar, but to granulation tissue in a healing wound before the formation of scar tissue.

9. 1: See Isaiah 38: 21 and I Timothy 5: 23.

9. 2: Isidore follows the traditional division of medicine into dietetics, drug therapy, and surgery; see Celsus, *De medicina*, Prooem. 9 and Pseudo-Soranus, *Quaestiones medicinales* 12 [Rose 249].

5. Every cure is brought about either by the use of contraries or by the use of similars. By contraries, as a chilling disease is treated with heat, or a dry one with moisture, just as also it is impossible for pride to be cured except it be cured by humility.

6. But by similars as a round dressing is applied to a round wound, or an oblong one to an oblong wound. Indeed, the bandages themselves are not the same for all wounds and for all members, but like is adapted to like, so that the two may assist each other, as their names imply.

7. For "antidote," *antidotum,* in Greek, is said in Latin "given from the contrary," for contraries are cured by contraries in the rationale of medicine, or alternatively, by a similar, as *PIKRA,* which is interpreted as "bitter," because it is bitter to the taste, deriving its name from similarity, since the bitter taste arising from diseases is usually dissolved by a bitter medication.

8. Every medication has been named for a reason proper to itself: some are called "holy," *hiera,* as though divine; expectorants, *arteriaca,* because they are suited to the windpipe, and alleviate swellings of the pharynx and air-passages. *Tiriaca* is an antidote against serpents by which their vena are warded off so that one poison is dissolved by the other. Cathartics, *catartica,* in Greek, are called purges, *purgatoria,* in Latin.

9. Pills, *catapotium,* [are so called] because only a small quantity is drunk or swallowed. *Diamoron* takes its name from the juice of the mulberry, *mora,* from which it is made, just as opium, *diacodion,* because [made] from *codia,* that is, from the poppy; just as *diaspermaton* because it is compounded from seeds.

10. An electuary, *electuarium,* is so named because it is sucked while soft. A troche, *trociscus,* is named because it is shaped like a little wheel: a wheel is called *TROCHOS* in Greek. Eyesalves, *collyrium,* are so named in Latin because they take away disorders of the eyes. A poultice, *epitima,* because superimposed

upon other things, it assists the medications already applied.

11. Poultices, *cataplasma,* are named because used to draw to a head; a plaster, *inplastrum,* because it is spread on; an emollient, *malagma,* because it is softened and compounded without the use of heat. *Enema* is a Greek name: in Latin, it is "an easing" *relaxatio.* Pessaries, *pessarium,* are named because they are inserted deep inside.

12. A certain Greek, Chiron, founded veterinary medicine: hence he is depicted as partly man and partly horse. Chiron, however, is named *APO TOU CHEIRIZESTHAI,* because he was a surgeon.

13. I believe that those days which the physicians term "critical," *creticus dies,* were so named because it is as though they sat in judgment over a man on such days concerning his illness, and by their sentence either punish him or set him free.

10. MEDICAL BOOKS

1. An aphorism, *aforismus,* is a short discussion describing the whole meaning of the subject proposed.

2. A prognostic, *prognostica,* is a forecast of illnesses, named from "knowing in advance," *praenoscere;* because it is necessary for the physician to know what has occurred in the past, to understand the present and to predict the future.

3. *Dinamidia,* "The Power of the Herbs," that is, their potency and powers, for the curative power itself in herbs is called *DUNAMIS;* whence also those books are named *dinamidia* in which their medical [values] are written.

4. A botany, *butanicum,* of herbs, is so called because therein the herbs are identified.

---

9. 5: The doctrine of therapy by "contraries" is based on the humoral pathology; see Pseudo-Soranus, *Quaestiones medicinales* 11 [Rose 248–249] and Galen, *Definitiones medicae* 9 [Kühn 19: 350–351].

9. 6: This passage suggests the ancient "doctrine of signatures," that nature designates the utility of medicinal plants by their external appearance.

9. 9–11: *Morus,* the mulberry, is mentioned at XVII. 7. 19 without comment on medicinal properties. Opium is described at XVII. 9. 31, see note 242 above. For a discussion of Roman pharmaceutical preparations, reflected in Isidore, see Celsus, *De medicina* 5. 17.

Collyria were, usually liquid, eyewashes or eyesalves, and there is a review of ancient ophthalmology at Paulus Aegineta, *Epitome* 3. 22. Enemata were used not only to empty the bowel, but for the administration of drugs, including cold water in fever; pessaries were not limited to gynecologic practice, but were usually lambs' wool soaked in various medications and introduced into a variety of bodily openings. See Celsus, *De medicina* 5. 21 for a thorough account of pessaries.

9. 12: See J. D. Gilruth, "Chiron and his Pupil Asclepius," *Annals of Medical History,* 3rd ser. 1 (1939): 158–176.

9. 13: The manuscripts read *creticos dies* quite consistently, and this is not to be confused with *criticos dies.* Acute infections, preeminently the pneumonias, may resolve by *lysis* or by *crisis. Lysis* is a gradual resolution of the fever and its associated illness, but *crisis* is a dramatic, abrupt change for the better: the fever breaks, the patient is bathed in sweat and there is marked improvement with promise of full recovery, often within a few hours. See Aurelius, *De acutis passionibus* 2 [Daremberg 492]; Celsus, *De medicina* 3. 4. 11; and Caelius Aurelianus, *De morbis acutis* 2. 36. At III. 7. 14–17, Isidore discusses the *dies canicularis,* which he thinks named from the dog star: purges are considered harmful on such days.

10. 3: On ancient herbals and books of materia medica, see L. C. MacKinney, " 'Dynamidia' in Medieval Medical Literature," *Isis* 24 (1936): 400–414, and C. J. Singer, "The Herbal in Antiquity," *Journal of Hellenic Studies* 47 (1927): 1–52. MacKinney feels that Isidore's definition is too restricted and reviews the subject in some detail.

11. PHYSICIANS' INSTRUMENTS

1. An instrument case, *enchiridion,* is named because it is carried in the hand, and contains many instruments, for the hand is called *CHEIR* in Greek.

2. The phlebotome, *phlebotomum,* is named from "incision," for in Greek, an incision is called *TOMÊ.*

3. Probe, *similarium* [. . .] Sharp hook, *angistrum* [. . .] Spatula-probe, *spatomele* [. . .] A cup, *guva,* is named by the Latins from its similarity to a gourd, *cucurbita;* from a sighing sound. When the vital spirit has been activated by a spark and when [the cup] has been placed over an incision into the body, everything either under the skin or deeper, which has been festering, whether humor or blood, is drawn to the surface.

4. Syringe, *clistere* [. . .] Pestles, *pila,* are named from pounding seeds [in a mortar], that is, grinding them. Hence also pigments, *pigmenta,* because they are handled with a pestle and mortar, as though PILIGMENTA. For a mortar, *pilum,* is a concave vessel fitted for use by physicians, in which they usually prepare barley-water, *ptisana,* and pound up drugs, *pigmenta.*

5. Varro reports that there was once in Italy a certain Pilumn[i]us, who was in charge of grinding grain, whence [also] are derived the names for miller and baker. The mortar and pestle by which grits, *far,* are ground were invented by him, and so are named after him. The pestle is that by which anything put into the mortar is ground.

6. A mortar, *mortarium,* is so called because those seeds which are put into it and which have been reduced to a powder are dead.

7. An eye-cup, *coticula,* is that in which liquid eye-salves, *collyrium,* which have been whirled about are applied. It is a delicate instrument since a coarse [instrument] would disperse the medication rather than prepare it for application.

12. BALSAMS AND UNGUENTS

1. Incense, *odor,* is named from air, *aër.*

2. Incense, *thymiama,* is named in the Greek language because it is fragrant, for thyme is the name of a flower which emits a perfume, concerning which Vergil [wrote] [*Georgics* 4. 169]: *redolentque thymo,* "And they smell of thyme."

3. Incense, *incensum,* is named because it is consumed by fire when it is offered.

4. *Tetraidos* are the oblong shapes for incense which is made from four ingredients: four in Greek is *TETTARA,* formula *EIDOS.*

5. Myrrh, *stacte,* is an incense which is squeezed out by pressure, and is named by the Greeks *PARA TO STAZEIN STAKTÊ,* that is, "crushed."

6. Balsam, *mirobalanum,* is named because it is made from a perfume-bearing nut, of which Horace wrote [*Odes* 3.29. 4]: *Et pressa tuis balanus capillis,* "And balsam pressed out for your hair." Oil, *oleum,* is pure and mixed with nothing else, but an unguent, *unguentum,* is anything made of common oil, fortified by an admixture with other kinds, taking on a pleasing and long-lasting odor.

7. Some unguents are named after places, as *telinum,* which Julius Caesar recalled, saying: *Corpusque suavi telino unguimus,* "And we anointed the body with sweet telinum." This was made on the Island of Telo, which is one of the Cyclades.

---

11. 1–3: For a discussion of ancient surgical instruments, usually brazen or steel, see J. A. Milne, *Surgical Instruments in Greek and Roman Times* (Oxford, 1907). Those mentioned by Isidore include:

(*a*) *Phlebotomum,* a bleeding lancet, used in many procedures other than venesection. Various sizes and shapes were made, fitted with sharp or guarded points, straight and curved blades, with single and double edges. The modern bistoury pointed scalpel most closely resembles the most typical ancient examples of this instrument. A similar knife was used by ancient scribes for the preparation of reed pens, the *SMILÊ* or medieval *scalpellum.*

(*b*) *Similarium* (or *specillum*), a probe or sound used in blunt dissection, but not for cutting tissue: *SMILÊ* is a scalpel, *MÊLÊ* a probe and *SMÊLÊ* seems to be a bastard form. This instrument was usually smaller than the

(*c*) *Spat(h)omele,* or spatula-probe. This consisted of a long shaft with an olive-shaped protuberance at one end and a spatula at the other. Originally a pharmacist's instrument, it found wide use as a probe, tongue-blade, meningophylax, cautery, and in blunt surgical dissection, examinations of internal orifices, and mixing drugs. Milne (p. 60) notes that the *nucleus,* or tip, averaged 7.5 mm. in diameter, the spatula 15 mm. in width, and the overall length 16 cm. in twenty surviving specimens examined by him.

(*d*) *Angistrum* (Greek *AGISTRON*), a sharp hook used both as a cutting instrument in various procedures and much as the modern surgeon used toothed forceps in handling tissue. Blunt hooks, without cutting edges and sometimes fitted with eyes like modern aneurysm needles, were often used to obtain hemostasis by traction on blood vessels, a procedure suggesting that ancient physicians may have had better ideas of blood circulation than we appreciate.

11. 3: See I. E. Drabkin, *Caelius Aurelianus on Acute Diseases and on Chronic Diseases* (Chicago, 1950), p. 51, for a note on cupping.

11. 4: *Clistere,* usually thought of as an enema syringe, was an instrument made of an animal bladder attached to a hollow tube. Such syringes were made in a variety of sizes for a variety of uses.

11. 7: *Coticula* generally was a small stone mortar for medical use, but Isidore's *citicula* (as in some manuscripts) is obviously an eyecup.

12. 5: Spengler has *APO TOU STAZEIN, quod est manare sive distillare,* but prefers to read *PARA TOU STAZESTHAI* and cites Horace, *Odes* 3. 29. 4. At Scribonius Largus, *Compositiones* 34, *stactor* is an eyewash, and at Celsus, *De medicina* 6. 7. F2, *stacten* is a species of myrrh favored by ophthalmologists.

12. 7: Otto and Spengler both derive *telinus* from the Greek *TÊLIS,* fenugreek, and ascribe the quotation in question to a play by one Strabo Tragicus and not to the Dictator.

8. Some also are named from their inventors, as *amaracinum:* some say that there was once a royal page named Amaracus, who was carrying many kinds of unguents when he chanced to fall, creating a better perfume from the mixture. For this reason, the very best perfumes are now called *amaracina;* actually, however, this comes from a species of flowers.

9. Likewise, there are others which are named [from] their kind, as rose [essence] from the rose, henna-oil from the flower henna, whence also [the name] refers to the scent of its active principle.

10. Of these, some are simple unguents made from one species only, whence the name and the perfume are the same, as *anetinum,* which is made simply from oil and anise, *anetum.* But some are made from a mixture of many ingredients, whence also they do not have the perfume which the name denotes, for they receive an undefined perfume from those elements which are mixed. Wax plaster, *cerotum* [. . .] Softening ointment, *calasticum* [. . .] Ointment, *marciatum* [. . .]

13. THE STUDY OF MEDICINE

1. Some ask why the art of medicine is not included among the other liberal disciplines. It is because whereas they embrace individual subjects, medicine embraces them all. The physician ought to know literature, *grammatica,* to be able to understand or to explain what he reads.

2. Likewise also rhetoric, that he may delineate in true arguments the things which he discusses; dialectic also so that he may study the causes and cures of infirmities in the light of reason. Similarly also

arithmetic, in view of the temporal relationships involved in the paroxysms of diseases and in diurnal cycles.

3. It is no different with respect to geometry because of the properties of regions and the locations of places. He should teach what must be observed in them by everyone. Moreover, music ought not be unknown by him, for many things are said to have been accomplished for ill men through the use of this art, as is said of David who cleansed Saul of an unclean spirit through the art of melody. The physician Asclepiades also restored a certain insane man to his pristine health through music.

4. Finally also, he ought to know astronomy, by which he should study the motions of the stars and the changes of the seasons, for as a certain physician said, our bodies are also changed with their courses.

5. Hence it is that medicine is called a second philosophy, for each discipline claims the whole of man for itself. Just as by philosophy the soul, so also by medicine the body is cured.

---

12. 9: *Quiprinum,* "henna oil," derived from the flower *quipro,* the henna, may be intended, but *quipro* may be a corruption of *ciprino* (see Caelius Aurelianus, *De morbis chronicis* 2. 4) which may be henna. Otto suggests, probably correctly, that *cypernum,* "cedar," is intended.

13. 3: Rudolf Allers, "Microcosmus," *Traditio* **2** (1944): 375–376, observes: "The relation between human music, inner harmony, and the harmony of the spheres, therefore the cosmic law, explains the high esteem in which music was held throughout medieval times."
Aristotle, *De caelo* 2. 9 [290b12] explains that man does not hear the music of the spheres since its sound is continuous, and man perceives sounds only when interrupted by periods of silence. Cassiodorus, *Institutes* 2. 5. 9, has a discussion of the medical usefulness of music.
13. 4: Cf. Hippocrates, *Airs, Waters and Places* 2: "Astronomy contributes not a little, but a very great deal indeed to medicine." There is a similar definition of the physician's propaideutic at Pseudo-Soranus, *Quaestiones medicinales,* Prooem. [Rose 244–245].
13. 5: The notion that philosophy, i.e., philosophical and metaphysical theology, would cure some of the disorders of the soul and the art of medicine some of those of the body developed early in Christian thought; see Tertullian, *De anima* 2. 6 [Waszink 4].

APPENDICES

A. "A NOTE ON THE PULSE"

Although the Hippocratic school seems to have paid less attention to the pulse in disease than post-classical Greco-Roman physicians (see Francis Adams, *The Genuine Works of Hippocrates* [London, 1849] 1: p. 351), there was extensive study of the changes in the pulse subsequent to the classical period. E. F. Horine ("An Epitome of Ancient Pulse Lore," *Bulletin of the History of Medicine* 10 [1941]: 209, at p. 211) notes:

Galen states that Herophilus was the first to describe the *pulsus caprizans*, an odd type with two phases, i.e., an initial stroke, thought to have been the result of imperfect dilatation of the artery, followed by a stronger one. This *pulsus caprizans*, also called *dorcadissans*, was said to resemble the leap of a goat (gazelle?) Herophilus is said by Pliny (A.D. 23–79) to have "reduced the pulses or beating of the arteries unto the times and measures in Musicke, according to the degrees of every age."

Francis Adams' translation of Paulus Aegineta, *Epitome* 2. 12 (*op. cit.* 1: pp. 202–213) provides an outline of the pulse lore common in post-classical medical practice after the time of Galen.

The pulse was studied and analyzed from ten carefully subdivided aspects: (1) *motion:* quick, slow, or moderate; broad, long, high, or deep; narrow, short, or low; (2) *character*, small or great; (3) *strength:* strong, weak, or moderate; (4) *consistency of the artery* (Galen's "tension"): hard, soft, or moderate; (5) *contents of the artery:* full, empty, or moderate; (6) *quality of heat in the heart;* (7) *time of rest:* dense, rare (that is, with a long interval of rest), or moderate—Adams compares this to the nineteenth-century "frequent" and "slow"; (8) *rhythm*, rhythmic or arrhythmic; (9) *regularity:* regular, that is, with equal periods of filling and emptying, or irregular; and (10) *equality:* whether equal or unequal. If the pulse were unequal, the following subdivisions were applied: (*a*) intermitting; (*b*) recurrent, with an extra beat; (*c*) sharp-tailed or *myuri* (= "mouse-tailed"); (*d*) failing or fainting *myuri;* (*e*) recurrent *myuri;* (*f*) *innuentes et circumnuentes*, a category hard to define, but probably "irregularly irregular"; (*g*) *dorcadissans*, a jerky pulse, rapid after intervals of rest and thought to characterize a febrile illness; (*h*) reverberating or *dicrotos*, a pulse which beats twice, the modern dicrotic pulse; (*i*) declining; (*j*) undulatory and vermicular; (*k*) spasmodic and vibratory; (*l*) *formicans* (= "antlike"), the smallest pulse, understood to indicate that the patient was dying; (*m*) hectic, a rapid pulse with little or no variation; (*n*) spasmodic, conveying the impression of a stretched cord; (*o*) vibratory; (*p*) serrated, a pulse suggesting to the palpating fingers that part of the artery is dilated and that part is not, or a pulse wherein part

of the artery appears harder than is natural; and (*q*) *dicrotos*, a small pulsation suddenly following or superimposed upon a larger pulsation. Thus, all of the possible disorders of the pulse had been recognized and named.

Galen divided the pulse into four parts: diastole and systole, separated by two periods of rest. The *pulsus dorcadizon* is discussed at Galen, *De pulsuum differentiis* 1. 28 [Kühn 8: 556] and the *pulsus formicans* at I. 26 [Kühn 8: 553]: these are the disordered pulses mentioned by Isidore at XI. 1. 120. At Pseudo-Soranus, *Quaestiones medicinales* 147–150 [Rose 263], the pulse is described. Diastole is the collapse and systole the filling of the artery due to the heart's action, and see Pseudo-Soranus, *Quaestiones medicinales* 183 [Rose 266] and 185 [Rose 266] for accounts which parallel XI. 1. 120.

B. "FRENESIS"

The limitations of ancient pathology were such that despite clinical descriptions of eminent clarity, symptoms were grouped to form disease entities: the analysis of symptoms superficially the same but due (e.g., jaundice) to widely different causes had to await a scientific pathologic anatomy and pathologic physiology. Thus, in Isidore as in ancient medical writers generally, *frenesis* is a general term applicable to mental disorientation accompanying many febrile illnesses. Celsus, *De medicina* 3. 18. 1 defines it as an acute insanity associated with fever. Psychiatric illness, roughly divided into mania and melancholia, was well known and described by ancient physicians, who were also familiar with the excitement induced by acute drug and alcoholic intoxication—mandrake root seems to have been a common offender among a certain population (see Caelius Aurelianus, *De morbis acutis* 1. 1–8). Since *frenesis* (or *phrenitis*, in some but not all cases) was associated with an acute febrile illness, it was rarely confused with a primary psychiatric illness or with epilepsy (see Caelius Aurelianus, *De morbis chronicis* 1. 5–6).

At Galen, *Definitiones medicae* 234 [Kühn 19: 412–413], *phrenitis* involves fever, disorientation, involuntary movement, and sometimes coma. Aurelius, *De acutis passionibus* 8 [Daremberg 692–693] gives a brief differential diagnosis between toxic or febrile and functional psychoses. Drug intoxication is not accompanied by fever, and the melancholy or psychotic patient has no fever although he speaks and acts strangely. The patient with *phrenitis* always has a fever, he is acutely ill, may develop pleuritis or pneumonia, and his disordered speech and behavior are associated only with the febrile illness. Pseudo-Soranus, *Quaestiones medicinales* 200 [Rose 268] gives a definition essentially that of Galen, *Definitiones medicae* 234. Cassius Felix, *De medicina* 62 [Rose 154] describes the appearance of a patient suffering from *frenesis*, and points out that this condition may occur not only with febrile illnesses but following a period of drunkenness (*vinolentia*): his description of a febrile, flushed patient with darting eyes, wakeful, moving about in bed, pulling at his bedclothes with complete mental disorientation and thready pulse is certainly *delirium tremens*.

Frenesis, then, was an acute toxic psychosis which might accompany any febrile illness, distinguished both from drug intoxications and acute psychotic reactions, but by no means limited to infections of the central nervous system as the more modern term *phrenitis* might suggest.

C. "THE ILIAC PASSION"

At IV. 6. 14, Lindsay suggests *EILISSEIN* as an emendation for †*ilios*† and see XI. 1. 100, and the note thereon above. An early eighth century manuscript (Wolfenbuttelanus Karolinus) has *ilea subvolvere;* Otto suggests *EILUEIN*, Arevalo *EILIEN* and various others *HEILISSEN*. Otto reads: *ileos dolor intestinorum. Unde et ilia dicta sunt. Graece enim EILUEIN obvolvere dicitur, quod se intestina prae dolore involvunt. Hi et torminosi dicuntur ab intestinorum tormento.*

Ileos, the "iliac disease" or "iliac passion" refers to what a modern surgeon has in mind when he speaks of "an acute abdomen," that is, a clinical syndrome marked by pain, vomiting, and abdominal distention resulting from one of a number of mechanical conditions which produce interruption of normal peristalsis, distention of a hollow viscus, and which have a potential for rupture and death, either from intestinal obstruction and its biochemical complications or peritonitis. A strict translation of *tormentum* as "twisted" is probably not justified except in so far as it refers to intussusception, with telescoping of a loop of intestine upon itself, or to strangulation of a hernia or of a portion of intestine: these conditions would require, ordinarily, laparotomy or autopsy for diagnosis.

Ileos, at Caelius Aurelianus, *De morbis acutis* 3. 17, includes acute intestinal obstruction from any cause: strangulation of a hernia, volvulus, fecal impaction, and obstruction by a tumor mass as well as intussusception, and may be the result of homicidal poisoning. His list of symptoms includes constipation, thirst, pain, and fever which end with fecal vomiting, collapse, and death. At Celsus, *De medicina* 2.1.8, *ileon* is Isidore's *lienteria* (IV. 7. 37), but at 4. 22. 1, he translates *STROPHOI* as *tormina*, which he refers to dysentery. Thomas Sydenham (*Opera Omnia*, ed. W. A. Greenhill [London, 1844], p. 160) characterizes the 1669 London epidemic of cholera as marked by *immania ventris tormina sine dejectionibus,* and the ancient *ileos*

may have included some cases of cholera. Isidore's *ileus* is certainly that of Caelius Aurelianus. *Chordapsus* is a synonym for *ileus*, and Cassius Felix, *De medicina* 51 [Rose 131–132] describes, as *ileos*, a syndrome characteristic of fatal peritonitis.

D. "A NOTE ON THE PLAGUE"

It has often been suggested that the term *bubonic* applied to the plague, which in ancient times may or may not have been the epidemic disease now produced by *P. pestis*, is derived from *bubes*, a late Latin consonantal corruption from *pubes*, and refers to the primary suppurative lesion in the inguinal lymph nodes which often marks the onset of this form of plague. *Bubo* has the same derivation. That plague might also be pulmonic may not have been appreciated by the ancients, assuming that the disease was the same, and the differentiation between an acute pneumonia (such as that frequently a fatal episode during the pandemic influenza of 1919–1920) and a disease as terrifying as epidemic plague would have been difficult. Francis Adams discusses the plague in his edition of Paulus Aegineta (*op. cit.*, 1: pp. 278–288).

There is a more extended discussion of plague at Isidore, *De natura rerum* 39 (Jacques Fontaine, ed., *Isidore de Séville: Traité de la Nature* [Bordeaux, 1960], pp. 303–305:

Plague is a disease which ravages widely and which infects almost all those whom it touches with its contagion. This illness does not even allow so much time as that in which to hope either for life or for death, but a feeling of weakness comes on very suddenly, bringing death at the same time. As to the true cause of this pestilence, someone has said, "Whenever for the sins of man a scourge and a chastening is laid upon the lands, then from any cause— that is, either from the force of dryness or heat or intemperance of rains—the air is corrupted. Thus, the elements are spoiled by a disturbed balance of the natural order; a corruption of the air arises, and a pestiferous exhalation develops, a power for corruption against men and other living things." Whence Vergil [*Aeneid* 3. 138–139] has said: *From a tainted part of the sky there came a pestilence for the wasting of our bodies and the unhappy ruin of trees.* Likewise, others say that many pest bearing seeds of things are carried into the air and borne up, then are transported either by winds or by clouds to the farthest parts of the heavens. Then, wherever they are carried, either they fall through our pores and joined together, encompass the beginnings of death for animals, or they remain suspended in the air, and when we breathe, we take in air, absorbing them at the same time into the body, then, falling ill, the body is extinguished either by foul ulcers or as though by a sudden blow. For just as bodies exposed to this unusual state of the heavens or unwholesomeness of the waters take the disease, so also corrupted air coming from other parts of the heavens snatch up the body with a sudden blow and quickly extinguish life.

See Clement, *Recognitiones* 8. 45 [*PG* 1: 1392] and Lucretius, *De rerum natura* 6. 1090–1102, 1119–1124. Although Arevalo refers IV.6.19 to Paul the Deacon, *De inguinaria nova Italiae peste ante Justini-*

anum, there is enough verbal similarity between Isidore, Pseudo-Clement, and Lucretius to suggest that Isidore may have compiled his account from them, depending upon Lucretius for his scientific hypothesis, which he Christianizes—so to speak—by reference to what was accepted in his day as a genuine writing by one of the most respected of the Greek fathers. The influence of prevailing winds on the plague is discussed by Isidore at XIII. 11. 6.

E. "A NOTE ON UNDULANT FEVERS"

Etymologiae IV. 7. 10 refers to *typi*, a group of fevers which probably resembled typhoid, malaria, and various undulant fevers now extinct or unidentifiable. In ancient clinical discussions of fever, four stages are commonly identified:

Beginning .... *Initium* ..... *ARCHĒ, APHORMĒ*
Increasing phase .. *Augmentum* .. *AUXĒSIS, EPIDOSIS*
Highest stage ... *Status* .... *AKMĒ*
Decline .... *Declinatio* ... *ANESIS, PARAKMĒ*

These stages are simply defined at Pseudo-Soranus, *Quaestiones medicinales* 88 [Rose 257] and at Galen, *Definitiones medicae* 136 [Kühn 19: 388] : the names of these stages of a febrile illness are self-explanatory. Their actual time sequence would vary from disease to disease, and would be helpful both in differential diagnosis and in predicting the outcome of any particular patient's case; contrast, e.g., the differing fever patterns between an acute bacterial pneumonia and a chronic tuberculous abscess. Ancient physicians attached great importance to the exact numerical relationships involved, and this is one of the reasons why Isidore felt (IV. 13. 2) that the physician should study mathematics.

The ancient *typhus* (the word *TUPHOS* is conventionally derived from the smoke of a burning funeral pyre: the *Iliad* begins during such an epidemic) was apparently a collective term which included several kinds of fevers accompanied by stupor and insensibility at some time during their course or termination. The *typi* which Isidore describes seem to be intermittent or remittent fevers, and although it is now impossible to identify them, the regular paroxysms of malaria would certainly suggest some relationship. Aurelius, *De acutis passionibus* 1 [Daremberg 489] describes the stages of a fever: the beginning is marked by moderate subjective awareness of fever; the increasing phase leads to the highest stage, which varies in duration and character from disease to disease and which increases until the beginning of the decline, unless the patient dies. There are periodic fevers which return daily, or every third or fourth day, and Aurelius' description clearly refers to quartan and tertian malaria.

Pseudo-Soranus, *Quaestiones medicinales* 125 [Rose 261] has much the same account of quotidian, tertian, and quartan malarial fevers. Active tuberculosis often has a daily fever spike and was certainly very common in ancient times. If Isidore's reference to herbs which grow in water (IV. 7. 10) can be stretched to imply that there is a relationship between the *typi*, or undulant or remittent fevers, and the marshy waters, the identification of these *typi* as malarial would be stronger, but this is conjectural. *Causus* was a very acute fever accompanied by thirst, diarrhea, vomiting, and a weak pulse, especially common in summer at Pseudo-Soranus, *Quaestiones medicinales* 113 [Rose 260]: this may or may not be cholera, since the *cholerae rejectione abundanter* refers to nothing more precise than bile-stained vomiting. The same writer, *Quaestiones medicinales* 120 [Rose 260–261] makes a good case for something like typhoid fever, with a "marshy" odor and a slow, weak pulse (*AMUDRON*, "dim," "faint") and a cold, foul-smelling perspiration. He terms this *typhodes febris*.

BIBLIOGRAPHY

A. Texts

ANSPACH, EDUARD. 1930. *Taionis et Isidori nova fragmenta et opera* (Madrid).

AREVALO, FAUSTINUS. 1797–1803. *Isidori Hispalensis opera omnia denuo correcta et aucta* (Rome; reprinted in Migne, *Patrologia latina* 81–84).

BECKER, GUSTAVUS, ed. 1857. *Isidori Hispalensis de natura rerum liber* (Berlin).

BEER, RUDOLF. 1909. *Etymologiae: codex Toletanus (nunc Matritensis) 15. 8 phototypice editus* (Leyden).

DOLD, ALBAN. 1940. "Irische Isidorfragmente des 7. Jhs," *Texte und Arbeiten herausgegeben durch die Erzabtei Beuron* 31 (Beuron).

FONTAINE, JACQUES. 1960. *Isidore de Séville: Traité de la nature* (Bordeaux).

LINDSAY, W. M., ed. 1911. *Isidori Hispalensis episcopi Etymologiarum sive originum libri XX* (Oxford).

OTTO, F. V., ed., 1833. *Isidori Hispalensis etymologiarum libri*, in Lindemann, J. F., ed., *Corpus grammaticorum latinorum veterum* (Leipzig), 3.

SCHWARZ, HEINRICH. 1895. *Observationes criticae in Isidori Hispalensis origines* (Hirschberg).

B. Sources

ADAMS, FRANCIS. 1844–1847. *The Seven Books of Paulus Aegineta Translated from the Greek* (London).

DAREMBERG, CHARLES. 1846. "Aurelius de acutis passionibus," *Janus* 2: 468–499, 690–696, 706–731.

—— 1879. *Rufus d'Éphèse: Œuvres* (Paris).

DETLEFSEN, D., ed. 1866–1882. *C. Plinii secundi naturalis historia* (Berlin).

DRABKIN, I. E. 1950. *Caelius Aurelianus on Acute diseases and on Chronic Diseases* (Chicago).

GOETZ, GEORGE, and FREDERICK SCHOELL, eds. 1910. *M. Terenti Varronis de lingua latina quae supersunt* (Leipzig).

HELMREICH, GEORGE, ed. 1887. *Scriboni Largi Conpositiones* (Leipzig).

HOWALD, ERNEST, and H. E. SIGERIST, eds. 1927. *Antonii Musae de herba vettonica liber; Pseudoapulei herbarius; Anonymi de taxone liber; Sexti Placiti liber medicinae ex animalibus* (Leipzig and Berlin).

KENT, R. G. 1938. *Varro on the Latin language with an English translation* (London).

MYNORS, R. A. B., ed. 1937. *Cassiodori Senatoris Institutiones* (Oxford).

ROSE, VALENTINE. 1870. *Anecdota graeca et graecolatina* (Berlin) 2: Pseudo-Soranus, *Quaestiones medicinales*, pp. 241–280; Soranus, *Responsiones medicinales*, pp. 161–240.

—— ed. 1875. *Plinii secundi quae fertur una cum Gargilii Martialis medicina nunc primum edita* (Leipzig).

—— ed. 1879. *Cassii Felicis de medicina ex Graecis logicae sectae auctoribus liber* (Leipzig).

SPENCER, W. G. 1935–1938. *Celsus de medicina with an English translation* (Cambridge, Massachusetts).

WASZINK, J. H., ed. 1947. *Quinti Septimi Florentis Tertulliani de anima* (Amsterdam).

C. Authorities

ALLBUTT, T. C. 1901. *Science and Medieval Thought* (London).

—— 1922. *Greek Medicine in Rome* (London).

ARIAS, IRENE A., ANTONIO TOVAR, and A. R. MORENO. 1950. *La medicina en la obra de san Isidoro* (Buenos Aires).

BAREILLE, G. 1924. "Isidore de Séville," *Dictionnaire de Théologie Catholique* (Paris) 8: 98–111.

BEESON, C. H. 1913. "Isidor-Studien," *Quellen und Untersuchungen zur Lateinischen Philologie des Mittelalters* (Munich) 4, No. 2.

[CAMACHO, D. B., and C. E. ARQUÉS]. 1945. *Isidori Hispalensis Ethimologiae IIII: De medicina* (Barcelona).

BREHAUT, ERNEST. 1912. *An Encyclopedist of the Dark Ages: Isidore of Seville* (New York).

BROWN, R. B. 1949. *The Printed Works of Isidore of Seville* (Lexington, Kentucky).

CAÑAL, CARLOS. 1897. *San Isidoro: esposición de sus obras* (Seville).

COCHRANE, C. N. 1940. *Christianity and Classical Culture* (New York).

CORTÉS Y GONGORA, LUIS. 1951. *Etimologías: versión castellana* (Madrid).

GRAHAM, E. K. 1934. *The De Universo of Hrabanus Maurus* (Chapel Hill: typescript A. M. thesis, University of North Carolina).

D'IRSAY, STEPHEN. 1927. "Patristic Medicine," *Annals of Medical History* 9: 364–378.

—— 1928. "An Historical Dictionary of Medicine," *Kyklos* 1: 157–159.

—— 1930. "Christian Medicine and Science in the Third Century," *The Journal of Religion* 10: 515–544.

DRESSEL, ENRICO. 1874–1875. "De Isidori Originum fontibus," *Rivista di filologia e d'Istruzione Classica* 3: 207–268.

D'AULT-DUMESNIL, E. 1843. "Etude sur la vie, les œuvres, et les temps de St. Isidore de Séville," *L'Université Catholique* 16: 145–157, 352–367.

FLETCHER, G. R. J. 1919. "St. Isidore of Seville and his Book on Medicine," *Proceedings of the Royal Society of Medicine, Section of the history of medicine* 12: 70–95.

FONTAINE, JACQUES. 1959. *Isidore de Séville et la culture classique dans l'espagne wisigothique* (Paris).

HARNACK, ADOLF. 1892. *Medicinisches aus der Ältesten Kirchengeschichte* (Leipzig).

HOMEYER, GEORG. 1913. *De scholiis Vergilianis Isidori fontibus* (Jena).

KÄSTNER, H. F. 1896. "Pseudo-Dioscorides de herbis femininis," *Hermes* 31: 578–636.

KETTNER, H. 1865. *Varronische studien* (Halle).

KIBRE, PEARL. 1945. "Hippocratic Writings in the Middle Ages," *Bulletin of the History of Medicine* 18: 371–412.

KLUSSMANN, M. 1892. *Excerpta Tertulliana in Isidori Hispalensis Etymologiis* (Hamburg).

KÜBLER, B. 1890. "Isidorusstudien," *Hermes* 25: 496–526.

LAISTNER, M. L. W. 1935. "The Christian Attitude to Pagan Literature," *History* 20: 49–54.

—— 1957. *The Intellectual Heritage of the Early Middle Ages* (Ithaca).

—— 1957. *Thought and Letters in Western Europe, A.D. 500–900* (2nd ed., London).

LINDSAY, W. M. 1911. "The Editing of Isidore 'Etymologiae'," *The Classical Quarterly* 5: 42–53.

—— 1924. "Note on the Use of Glossaries for the Dictionary of Medieval Latin," *Bulletin du Cange* 1: 16.

LEAR, F. S. 1936. "St. Isidore and Mediaeval Science," *The Rice Institute Pamphlet* 23: 75–105.

LOT, FERDINAND. 1931. "A Quelle Époque a-t-on cessé de parler Latin," *Bulletin du Cange* 6: 97.

LYNCH, C. H. 1938. *Saint Braulio, Bishop of Saragossa (631–651): his life and writings* (Washington).

MACKINNEY, L. C. 1937. *Early Mediaeval Medicine with Special Reference to France and Chartres* (Baltimore).

—— 1938. "Medieval Medical Dictionaries and Glossaries," *Medieval and Historiographical Studies in Honor of James Westfall Thompson* (Chicago).

MAITRE, LÉON. 1924. *Les Écoles Épiscopales et monastiques en occident avant les universités* (2nd ed., Paris).

Miscellanea Isidoriana . . . en el XIII centenario de su muerte (Rome, 1936).

NETTLESHIP, HENRY. 1885. *Lectures and Essays on Subjects Connected with Latin Literature and Scholarship* (Oxford).

—— 1895. *Lectures and Essays: Second Series* (Oxford).

PROBST, OTTO. 1915. "Isidors Schrift 'de Medicina'," *Archiv für Geschichte der Medizin* 8: 22–38.

PUHLMANN, WALTER. 1930. "Die lateinische medizinische Literatur des frühen Mittelalters: Ein bibliographischer Versuch," *Kyklos* 3: 395–416.

SARTON, GEORGE. 1927. *Introduction to the History of Science* (Washington) 1.

SCHENK, ARNO. 1909. *De Isidori Hispalensis de rerum natura libelli fontibus* (Jena).

SCHNEIDER, DR. 1843. "Noch ein Wort über Magnentius Rabanus Maurus," *Janus* 2: 125–131.

SIGERIST, H. E. 1934. "The Medical Literature of the Early Middle Ages," *Bulletin of the Institute of the History of Medicine* 2: 26–50.

—— 1941. "Medieval Medicine," *University of Pennsylvania Bicentennial Conference, Studies in the History of Science* (Philadelphia).

—— 1958. "The Latin Medical Literature of the Early Middle Ages," *Journal of the History of Medicine* 13: 127–146.

SPENGLER, L. 1848. "Isidorus Hispalensis in seiner Bedeutung für die Naturwissenschaften und Medicin," *Janus* 3: 54–90.

STAHL, W. H. 1962. *Roman Science: Origins, Development, and Influence* (Madison).

SUDHOFF, KARL. 1916. "Die verse Isidors auf dem Schrank der medizinischen Werke seiner Bibliothek," *Mitteilungen zur Geschichte der Medizin* 15: 200–204.

THORNDIKE, LYNN. 1929. *A History of Magic and Experimental Science During the First Thirteen Centuries of Our Era* (London).

VOSSLER, KARL. 1948. "Isidorus von Sevilla," *Aus der Romanischen Welt* (Karlsruhe), pp. 551–562.

INDEX

70

www.ingramcontent.com/pod-product-compliance
Lightning Source LLC
Chambersburg PA
CBHW081334190326
41458CB00018B/5993